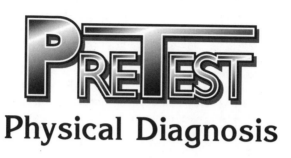

Physical Diagnosis

PreTest®
Self-Assessment
and Review

Notice

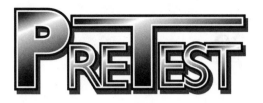

Physical Diagnosis

PreTest® Self-Assessment and Review

Third Edition

Editor

Tyson K. Cobb, M.D.
Orthopaedic Clinic of Mt. Vernon
Mt. Vernon, Illinois

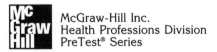

McGraw-Hill Inc.
Health Professions Division
PreTest® Series

New York • St. Louis • San Francisco • Auckland • Bogotá
Caracas • Lisbon • London • Madrid • Mexico City • Milan • Montreal
New Delhi • San Juan • Singapore • Sydney • Tokyo • Toronto

McGraw-Hill

*A Division of The **McGraw·Hill** Companies*

Physical Diagnosis: PreTest® Self-Assessment and Review, Third Edition
Copyright © 1998 1995 1992 by The McGraw-Hill Companies, Inc. All rights
reserved. Printed in the United States of America.

1 2 3 4 5 6 7 8 9 0   DOCDOC   9 9 8 7

ISBN 0-07-052531-5

The editors were John Dolan and Bruce MacGregor.
The production supervisor was Helene G. Landers.
Cover Designer was Jim Sullivan / RepoCat Graphics & Editorial Services.
R.R. Donnelley & Sons was printer and binder.
This book was set in Times Roman by V&M Graphics.

Library of Congress Cataloging-in-Publication Data

Physical diagnosis : PreTest self-assessment and review / edited by
  Tyson K. Cobb. — 3rd ed.
      p.   cm.
  Includes bibliographical references.
  ISBN 0-07-052531-5
  1. Physical diagnosis—Examinations, questions, etc. I. Cobb,
Tyson K.
  [DNLM: 1. Diagnosis—examination questions.   2. Physical
Examination—examination questions.   WB 18.2 P5775 1998]
RC76.P5   1998
616.07′54′076—dc21
DNLM/DLC
for Library of Congress   97-10550
                                              CIP

To my family
for their unselfish support of my academic endeavors
T.K.C.

Contents

Acknowledgments

The editor expresses gratitude to the following contributors:

Matthew D. Barrows, M.D.
Karen Gremminger Bullard, M.D.
Stephen Mark Bullard, M.D.
Albert C. Cuettar, M.D.
Martha Louise Elks, M.D., Ph.D.
Anne C. Epstein, M.D.
Joseph W. Kraft, M.D.
Gerald S. Laros II, M.D.

Thomas J. Motycka, M.D.
Kenneth H. Neldner, M.D.
Carl Thomas Nichols, M.D.
J. Rush Pierce, Jr., M.D.
Douglas R. Shelton, M.D.
Scott A. Smith, M.D.
Robert S. Urban, M.D.

Introduction

Physical Diagnosis: PreTest® Self-Assessment and Review, 3/e, has been designed to provide medical students, as well as physicians, with a comprehensive and convenient instrument for self-assessment and review of physical diagnosis. The 500 questions provided have been designed to parallel the format and degree of difficulty of the questions contained in the United States Medical Licensing Examination (USMLE) Step 1 and Step 2.

Each question in the book is accompanied by an answer, a paragraph explanation, and a specific page reference to a current journal article, a textbook, or both. A bibliography that lists all the sources used in the book follows the last chapter.

Perhaps the most effective way to use this book is to allow yourself one minute to answer each question in a given chapter; as you proceed, indicate your answer beside each question. By following this suggestion, you will be approximating the time limits imposed by the board examinations previously mentioned.

When you have finished answering the questions in a chapter, you should then spend as much time as you need verifying your answers and carefully reading the explanations. Although you should pay special attention to the explanations for the questions you answered incorrectly, you should read every explanation. The authors of this book have designed the explanations to reinforce and supplement the information tested by the questions. If, after reading the explanations for a given chapter, you feel you need still more information about the material covered, you should consult and study the references indicated.

General Appearance of Disease

DIRECTIONS: Each item below contains a question or incomplete statement followed by suggested responses. Select the **one best** response to each question.

1. A 15-year-old boy presents with complaints of pain in the left hip. The pain has been present for approximately 3 weeks and is increasing in severity. It is worse at night and is relieved by aspirin. There is no history of trauma or previous hip problems. This history is most consistent with

(A) osteoarthritis
(B) septic joint
(C) osteoid osteoma
(D) avascular necrosis
(E) muscle strain

2. All the following would be typical presenting signs or symptoms of *early* septic shock EXCEPT

(A) flushed appearance
(B) warmth
(C) elevated cardiac output
(D) agitation
(E) obtundation

3. Which of the following would be LEAST likely to be associated with gastrointestinal bleeding?

(A) Hypotension and tachycardia
(B) Ingestion of nonsteroidal anti-inflammatory agents
(C) History of prior gastrointestinal bleeding
(D) Alcohol abuse
(E) Negative stool guaiac testing

4. All the following signs and symptoms are consistent with *early* compartment syndrome of the flexor compartment of the forearm EXCEPT

(A) pain disproportionate to what might be expected for the degree of injury
(B) unrelenting pain after a pain-free interval
(C) pain with passive finger extension
(D) a swollen and tense flexor compartment
(E) loss of the radial pulse at the wrist and of motor function

5. Which of the following best describes a third-degree sprain?

(A) An injury that results in fracture of bone at the site of ligament attachment
(B) Ankle pain with ambulation
(C) A complete tear of a ligament that results in joint instability
(D) A tear of a minimum number of ligamentous fibers with tenderness but no instability
(E) A tear of a greater number of ligamentous fibers with loss of function and joint reaction but no instability

6. Cushing's syndrome is characterized by all the following EXCEPT

(A) hirsutism
(B) truncal obesity
(C) hyperpigmentation of buccal mucosa
(D) poor wound healing
(E) acne

7. A 3½-year-old girl is brought to your office by her parents who are concerned about her knock-knees (genu valgum). The parents state she was bowlegged as an infant and has become progressively knock-kneed over the past 6 months. The patient is otherwise healthy and has met all developmental milestones. Height and weight are within the 80th percentile. The femoral-tibial angle measures 14 degrees bilaterally. The intramalleolar distance is 10 cm with the knees just touching. The most likely diagnosis is

(A) Blount's disease
(B) physiologic knock-knees
(C) malunion
(D) rickets
(E) partial physeal arrest

8. A 17-month-old boy is found to have multiple fractures and blue sclerae. This is most characteristic of

(A) osteogenesis imperfecta
(B) osteoporosis
(C) achondroplasia
(D) osteomalacia
(E) osteitis deformans

9. A 21-year-old man presents to the office for a sore throat. On examination, the patient is found to be tall, with gynecomastia and testicular atrophy. Which is the most likely diagnosis?

(A) Testicular feminization syndrome
(B) 45,X (Turner's syndrome)
(C) Trisomy 21 (Down's syndrome)
(D) 47,XXY (Klinefelter's syndrome)
(E) Hepatic cirrhosis

10. Arthritis, fatigue, and a malar rash would most likely be associated with which of the following?

(A) Psoriasis
(B) Pseudogout
(C) Systemic lupus erythematosus (SLE)
(D) Rheumatoid arthritis
(E) Osteoarthritis

11. Seven light-brown maculae, each greater than 1 cm in diameter on the trunk of a patient with axillary freckling and firm subcutaneous masses, would suggest the diagnosis of

(A) Peutz-Jeghers syndrome
(B) tuberous sclerosis
(C) Sturge-Weber syndrome
(D) Albright's disease
(E) neurofibromatosis

12. A patient who is tall for her age and has long fingers and lenticular dislocation would likely have which of the following associated symptoms?

(A) A marked decrease in joint mobility
(B) Mitral valve prolapse or an aortic aneurysm
(C) Shortness of breath
(D) Dermal hemorrhage
(E) A negative thumb sign (Steinberg's sign)

13. All the following statements are true of the pivot shift test EXCEPT

(A) the pivot shift test is used to diagnose anterior cruciate ligament deficiency of the knee
(B) the posterior pull of the iliotibial tract is responsible for the reduction observed during this test
(C) the phenomenon observed during this test is due to rotational forces
(D) an internal rotational force is applied to the foot/leg during this test
(E) a valgus stress is applied to the knee during this test

14. Which of the following best describes the term *arthritis*?

(A) Any inflammatory process in a joint
(B) Deterioration of articular cartilage
(C) Joint infection
(D) Any disease of the joint
(E) Joint pain

15. When performing a physical examination, all the following are true EXCEPT

(A) Weber's test may help distinguish sensory from conductive hearing loss
(B) inspection of the chest should precede auscultation
(C) inspection of hands and nails may provide clues about respiratory problems
(D) intraocular pressure is best determined by the examination of retinal vessels
(E) the Snellen chart is used to test visual acuity

16. All the following statements concerning measurement of axillary temperature as opposed to oral or rectal temperature in a pediatric patient are true EXCEPT

(A) oral temperature is difficult to take in young children who do not understand instructions
(B) in a frightened child, insertion of an instrument into the rectum will serve to increase anxiety
(C) axillary temperature is usually more than 0.5°C lower than oral temperature
(D) axillary temperature can be determined more rapidly than oral or rectal temperature
(E) rectal temperature is the most accurate of the above three methods for assessing body temperature

17. Which of the following statements is true concerning the measurement of blood pressure?

(A) The bladder should encircle approximately 80 percent of the circumference of the limb
(B) A cuff that is too wide will give an artificially high reading
(C) Readings from the two arms generally vary by more than 20 mmHg in a normal patient
(D) It is not necessary to fully deflate the cuff before repeating a measurement
(E) The pressure at which Korotkoff sounds disappear should be read as the systolic pressure

18. Fullness of the infracondylar recess just inferior to the lateral condyle of the humerus would be consistent with all the following EXCEPT

(A) subluxation of the ulnar nerve
(B) effusion of the elbow joint
(C) synovitis
(D) dislocation of the radial head
(E) fracture of the radial head

19. Which of the following involves a partial tear of a musculotendinous unit?

(A) Fracture
(B) First-degree strain
(C) Second-degree strain
(D) Third-degree strain
(E) Contusion

20. A clinical feature that aids in making the diagnosis of pityriasis rosea is the fact that

(A) Wickham's striae are present
(B) the lesions recur frequently
(C) lesions follow skin cleavage lines
(D) the disease is communicable
(E) dramatic improvement follows administration of tetracycline

21. The sensitivity of digital rectal examinations can be characterized as

(A) high for rectal carcinoma and prostate carcinoma
(B) high for prostate carcinoma but low for appendicitis
(C) high for appendicitis and prostate carcinoma
(D) low for appendicitis, prostate carcinoma, and rectal carcinoma
(E) low for prostate carcinoma and high for rectal carcinoma

22. A patient presents with an osteoma of the jaw. Other signs or symptoms that might lead to the diagnosis of Gardner's syndrome include

(A) rapidly enlarging bones in both hands
(B) hematuria
(C) exophthalmos
(D) colonic polyps
(E) lytic skull lesions seen on x-ray

23. A child with Sprengel's deformity would most likely demonstrate all the following EXCEPT

(A) limited abduction of the shoulder
(B) limited internal rotation of the shoulder
(C) elevation of one shoulder
(D) loss of the normal contour of the neck
(E) a neck that appears full on one side

DIRECTIONS: The group of questions below consists of lettered options followed by numbered items. For each numbered item, select the appropriate lettered option(s). Each lettered option may be used once, more than once, or not at all. **Choose exactly the number of options indicated following each item.**

Items 24–27

Match each symptom or sign with the appropriate disease.

(A) Sjögren's syndrome
(B) Systemic lupus erythematosus
(C) Rheumatoid arthritis
(D) Ankylosing spondylitis
(E) Psoriatic arthropathy

24. Stiff back in the morning that improves with exercise **(SELECT 1 DISEASE)**

25. Skin lesions **(SELECT 1 DISEASE)**

26. Dry eyes and dry mouth **(SELECT 1 DISEASE)**

27. Butterfly rash **(SELECT 1 DISEASE)**

Items 28–31

Match each sign or set of signs with the appropriate syndrome.

(A) Down's syndrome
(B) Turner's syndrome
(C) Edwards' syndrome
(D) Patau's syndrome
(E) Klinefelter's syndrome

28. Epicanthal folds, broad nose, protruding tongue **(SELECT 1 SYNDROME)**

29. Testicular atrophy **(SELECT 1 SYNDROME)**

30. Short female with a webbed neck **(SELECT 1 SYNDROME)**

31. Prominent occiput, micrognathia, cleft lip and palate **(SELECT 1 SYNDROME)**

Items 32–35

Match each clinical picture with the appropriate arthropod.

(A) *Ornithodoros coriaceus* (pajaroello tick)
(B) *Latrodectus mactans* (black widow spider)
(C) *Dermacentor andersoni* (Rocky Mountain wood tick)
(D) *Loxosceles reclusa* (brown recluse spider)
(E) *Trombicula larvae* (chiggers)

32. Central necrotic area expanding in size up to 20 cm **(SELECT 1 ARTHROPOD)**

33. Weakness in the legs followed by ascending flaccid paralysis **(SELECT 1 ARTHROPOD)**

34. Pruritic papules or papulourticarial lesions persisting for days to weeks **(SELECT 1 ARTHROPOD)**

35. Intense muscle pains, abdominal rigidity, and nausea **(SELECT 1 ARTHROPOD)**

Items 36–39

Match each skin manifestation with the appropriate cause.

(A) Chronic arsenic ingestion
(B) Viral hepatitis
(C) Melanism
(D) Rubella
(E) Quinacrine ingestion

36. Tanned skin even when there is no sun exposure **(SELECT 1 CAUSE)**

37. Yellow skin and yellow sclerae **(SELECT 1 CAUSE)**

38. Gray skin with dark maculae **(SELECT 1 CAUSE)**

39. Greenish-yellow skin **(SELECT 1 CAUSE)**

Items 40–43

Match each description or disease below with the correct ocular sign.

(A) Arcus senilis
(B) Kayser-Fleischer ring
(C) Pterygium
(D) Chalazion
(E) Blepharitis

40. Gray band of corneal opacity in a 25-year-old man with hyperlipidemia **(SELECT 1 SIGN)**

41. Wilson's disease **(SELECT 1 SIGN)**

42. Granulomatous cyst of a meibomian gland **(SELECT 1 SIGN)**

43. Vascular membrane growing toward center of cornea **(SELECT 1 SIGN)**

Items 44–50

For each finding, select the most appropriate diagnosis.

(A) Acute pancreatitis
(B) Perforated duodenal ulcer
(C) Nephrotic syndrome
(D) Hypothyroidism
(E) Alzheimer's disease
(F) Parkinson's disease
(G) Rubeola (measles)
(H) Varicella (chicken pox)

44. Partial alleviation of pain when the patient sits up and leans forward **(SELECT 1 DIAGNOSIS)**

45. Rebound tenderness and abdominal guarding **(SELECT 1 DIAGNOSIS)**

46. Koplik's spots **(SELECT 1 DIAGNOSIS)**

47. Superficial vesicles with erythematous bases **(SELECT 1 DIAGNOSIS)**

48. Shuffling gait **(SELECT 1 DIAGNOSIS)**

49. Dementia **(SELECT 2 DIAGNOSES)**

50. Coarse hair **(SELECT 1 DIAGNOSIS)**

General Appearance
of Disease
Answers

1. The answer is C. *(Wold, pp 2–7.)* A history of pain that increases in severity, worsens at night, and is relieved by aspirin should suggest osteoid osteoma as a potential diagnosis. It is three times more common in males. Patients in their second decade of life are most commonly affected. The proximal femur is the most common location. Osteoarthritis is a common cause of hip pain in elderly patients. A septic hip joint is typically very acute with other constitutional signs of infection. Only osteoid osteoma has a classic history of relief with aspirin.

2. The answer is E. *(Tintinalli, 4/e, p 201.)* The early phase of septic shock is characterized by vasodilation, resulting in a warm, flushed patient with normal or elevated cardiac output. Fever, agitation, or confusion is often present. In *late* septic shock, patients may be obtunded with decreased urine output, blood pressure, and cardiac output.

3. The answer is E. *(Tintinalli, 4/e, p 221.)* Patients with gastrointestinal bleeding may have a history of prior gastrointestinal bleeding, use of non-steroidal anti-inflammatory agents, alcohol abuse, or use of corticosteroids or anticoagulants. Vital signs will reveal hypotension and tachycardia if blood loss is significant. Guaiac stool testing is usually positive. Ingestion of iron or bismuth can simulate melena. Guaiac testing in this setting will be negative.

4. The answer is E. *(Rockwood, 4/e, pp 487–492.)* Compartment syndrome results from elevated pressure within a closed space. Irreversible damage to the contents of the compartment will occur if elevated pressures persist. This condition should be considered a surgical emergency. The most important symptom is pain disproportionate to what might be expected for the problem for which the patient is being treated. Patients may have a pain-free interval after an injury and then develop unrelenting pain. They may complain of numbness or tingling in the affected extremity. The compartment is tense and tender to palpation, and passive muscle stretch increases the pain. Loss of pulse and motor function are late signs of compartment syndrome. Irreversible damage has usually occurred by the time these latter two findings present.

5. The answer is C. *(Hoppenfeld, p 370.)* A sprain is an injury to a ligament. A first-degree sprain is a minor injury with no instability. A second-degree sprain is a more significant injury with tearing of a greater amount of ligamentous fibers but still no instability. A third-degree sprain results in a complete tear of the ligament with resultant joint instability. If the attachment site of a ligament is fractured, this is called a *sprain fracture* or *avulsion fracture.*

6. The answer is C. *(Isselbacher, 13/e, pp 1960–1965.).* Hyperpigmentation of the skin, particularly in areas with creases or scars, along with pigmentation of the buccal mucosa is seen in primary adrenocortical insufficiency. Hirsutism, truncal obesity, poor wound healing, and acne are some of the classic signs of hyperadrenocorticalism.

7. The answer is B. *(Morrissy, 4/e, pp 1055–1061.)* Physiologic bowleg occurs in the first 2 years of life. Lateral bowing of the tibia is seen in the first year and bowleg involving both the tibia and distal femur occurs during the second year. Physiologic knock-knee is most pronounced between 3 and 4 years of age. Physiologic variations are common and most resolve with time. Pathologic forms are uncommon and generally do not resolve. The physician should assess growth, nutrition, symmetry, degree of deformity, and other abnormalities. Blount's disease is tibia vara, which results from abnormal growth of the proximal medial physis and metaphysis. It is more common in blacks and obese children. Medial tibial torsion often accompanies the deformity. An asymmetric deformity with a history of trauma may suggest malunion or partial physeal arrest. Rickets should be suspected in a patient with progressive varus deformity whose stature is below the 5th percentile. The diagnosis is confirmed by a low calcium and phosphorus and high alkaline phosphatase activity.

8. The answer is A. *(Isselbacher, 13/e, p 2111.)* Osteogenesis imperfecta is inherited as an autosomal dominant trait. It is characterized by brittle bones and often presents with multiple pathologic fractures. Other characteristics include blue sclerae, short stature, deformed skull, hearing loss, and dental abnormalities.

9. The answer is D. *(Isselbacher, 13/e, pp 2041–2043.)* Persons with Klinefelter's syndrome have a 47,XXY karyotype and are typically tall and eunuchoid in appearance, with gynecomastia, testicular atrophy, and a female pattern of hair distribution. Patients with Turner's syndrome are 45,X or are mosaic and have a female phenotype. Trisomy 21 in either sex presents with characteristic facial features and invariable mental retardation. Testicular feminization syndrome results from defective or absent androgen receptors throughout the body. These patients are 46,XY, but have a female phenotype. Destruction of the liver parenchyma may take away a person's ability to fully metabolize endogenous estrogens and thus lead to gynecomastia and testicular atrophy. However, the young age of the patient and his eunuchoid appearance suggest a 47,XXY karyotype (Klinefelter's syndrome).

10. The answer is C. *(Isselbacher, 13/e, pp 1643–1648, 1698–1700.)* Arthritis or arthralgias are seen in 90 percent of patients with SLE. A patient is said to have SLE if any four of the following eleven criteria are found: (1) malar rash, (2) discoid rash, (3) photosensitivity, (4) oral ulcers, (5) arthritis, (6) serositis (pleuritis or pericarditis), (7) renal disorders (persistent proteinuria or cellular casts), (8) neurologic disorders (seizures or psychosis), (9) hematologic disorders (hemolytic anemia, leukopenia, lymphopenia, thrombocytopenia), (10) immunologic disorders (positive LE cell preparation, antibody to DNA), or (11) antinuclear antibody. Arthritic manifestations usually involve proximal interphalangeal (PIP) and metacarpophalangeal (MCP) joints of the hands, wrists, and knees.

Pseudogout is a disorder involving calcium pyrophosphate crystals in the joint space. Onset is usually rapid and involved joints are erythematous, swollen, warm, and painful. Acute attacks are usually confined to a single joint; the knee is the most common site. The diagnosis is established by finding typical crystals (weakly positive birefringence under compensated polarized light) and is supported by radiographic evidence of chondrocalcinosis.

11. The answer is E. *(Morrissy, 4/e, pp 190, 256–257, 307.)* Six or more café au lait spots on the trunk and extremities with two or more subcutaneous neurofibromas is diagnostic for neurofibromatosis. Albright's disease, or polyostotic fibrous dysplasia, often presents as three or more irregularly shaped café au lait spots found unilaterally on the buttocks or cervical region. Peutz-Jeghers syndrome presents with pigmentation around the mouth. Sturge-Weber syndrome is a congenital disorder characterized by facial angioma, seizures, and mental retardation.

12. The answer is B. *(Morrissy, 4/e, pp 122, 179–180. Sapira, p 83.)* Marfan's syndrome is a congenital disease affecting three connecting tissue systems: skeletal, cardiovascular, and ocular. Mitral valve prolapse or an aortic aneurysm would therefore be consistent with this diagnosis. These patients usually have a positive thumb sign: when the fingers are clenched over the thumb, the thumb protrudes beyond the ulnar margin of the hand. Their arm span is greater than their height and the distance from their pubis to the floor is greater than one-half their height.

13. The answer is C. *(Miller, p 10.)* The pivot shift test is performed with the patient supine and the leg extended. The foot is held in internal rotation, and a valgus stress is placed on the knee. Gradual flexion (20 to 30°) results in reduction of the anteriorly displaced tibia and subsequently an audible sound ("clunk"). The iliotibial tract (band) is responsible for the reduction of the tibia. Anterior displacement of the tibia is made possible by lack of an intact anterior cruciate ligament. The pivot shift is due to abnormal anterior translation of the tibia and is not a rotational phenomenon as once believed.

14. The answer is A. *(Hoppenfeld, pp 22, 23, 288.)* Arthritis is defined as an inflammatory process in a joint. Osteoarthritis is a common progressive joint disorder characterized by a deterioration of articular cartilage and reactive new bone formation in the subchondral and juxtaarticular regions. Septic arthritis is joint inflammation due to infection caused by pyogenic organisms. Arthrosis is any disease of the joint. Arthrodynia is a painful joint.

15. The answer is D. *(Isselbacher, 13/e, pp 99, 104–105, 112, 181–183.)* While increased intraocular pressure may cause abnormalities that are seen on funduscopic examination, tonometry is the method of choice for assessing intraocular pressure. The Schiotz tonometer is placed on the cornea and intraocular pressure can be determined by the amount of indentation it causes. Glaucoma should be suspected in patients with pressures greater than 21 mmHg. Weber's test is performed by placing a vibrating tuning fork on the patient's head and determining if there is lateralization of sound to one side. In examining the chest, inspection is performed first and auscultation last. Cyanosis of the hands and clubbing of the fingers indicate hypoxemia, which may be caused by respiratory disease. The Snellen chart is used routinely to determine the smallest object a person can see at a distance of 20 feet (6 meters).

16. The answer is D. *(Athreya, p 82.)* Measurement of axillary temperature alleviates the need to insert a thermometer into the mouth or rectum, which might prove difficult in a child who is very young, anxious, or uncooperative. Axillary temperature tends to be at least 0.5°C lower than oral or rectal temperature. However, the thermometer must be properly positioned in the axilla for at least 2 min to obtain an accurate reading. Even so, rectal temperature measurements remain the most accurate.

17. The answer is A. *(Seidel, 3/e, pp 64–65.)* A cuff that is too wide will give an artificially low reading; the opposite is true of a cuff that is too narrow. Thus it is important to choose a cuff that is appropriate for the size of the patient's limb. The cuff should always be fully deflated prior to a second measurement to prevent vascular congestion, which could result in an inaccurate reading. In a normal patient, readings between the two arms rarely vary by more than 10 mmHg. The pressure at which Korotkoff sounds disappear is read as the diastolic, not systolic, pressure.

18. The answer is A. *(Morrey, 2/e, pp 74–76.)* The ulnar nerve passes on the medial aspect of the elbow joint between the medial epicondyle and the olecranon. Anterior subluxation of the ulnar nerve may be elicited and palpated during elbow flexion in some patients with recurrent subluxation of the ulnar nerve. The intracondylar recess is located just inferior to the lateral condyle of the humerus. It is normally marked by a depression in the contour of the skin. However, a loss of depression or fullness may be observed in patients with an elbow effusion, synovitis, or fracture, subluxation, or dislocation of the radial head.

19. The answer is C. *(Hoppenfeld, pp 73, 130, 376.)* A strain is an injury to a musculotendinous unit. It can be classified as first-degree (minimal stretching), second-degree (partial tear), or third-degree (complete disruption). A fracture is a break or disruption in the continuity of bone. A contusion is a bruise or injury to the soft tissue in which the skin is not broken.

20. The answer is C. *(Lynch, 3/e, pp 273–276, 394.)* Pityriasis rosea is a self-limiting papulosquamous eruption that is not spread by direct transmission. Generalized eruptions, which form a Christmas tree-like pattern along skin cleavage lines, are preceded by a "herald plaque," which is often misdiagnosed as ringworm. The condition rarely recurs and its course is not altered by antibiotics. Wickham's striae are white, reticulated lines sometimes seen on the skin lesions of lichen planus.

21. The answer is B. *(Muris, Fam Pract 10:34, 1993.)* The rectal examination has been advocated for assessing lower gastrointestinal abdominal and urinary symptoms. While it may have some value in assessing appendicitis, the yield is very low. Likewise, the diagnostic yield for rectal carcinoma is low. Nevertheless, rectal examinations have been shown to be useful in patients presenting with rectal symptoms. The sensitivity and yield of digital rectal examination for prostate-related problems are high.

22. The answer is D. *(Isselbacher, 13/e, pp 225, 301, 1425, 1621–1622, 1943–1944.)* Gardner's syndrome is characterized by the triad of bone tumors, soft tissue tumors, and colonic polyposis. The colonic polyps may predispose the patient to colon cancer. Exophthalmos is classically associated with Graves' disease of the thyroid. Lytic lesions of the skull in an elderly patient are suggestive of multiple myeloma.

23. The answer is B. *(Carson, J Bone Joint Surg 63A:1199–1207, 1981.)* Sprengel's deformity is congenital elevation of the scapula due to failure of the normal caudal migration of the scapula. In this deformity the scapula is usually elevated 2 to 10 cm and adducted with its inferior pole medially rotated. The medial rotation results in an abnormal position of the superomedial angle of the scapula, which causes the ipsilateral side of the neck to appear fuller with loss of the normal contour. The rotation also causes the glenoid cavity to face downward. This rotation combined with a relatively fixed scapula limits abduction to less than 100° in 40 percent of the patients with this condition. External and internal rotation are normal.

24–27. The answers are 24-D, 25-E, 26-A, 27-B. *(Morrissy, 4/e, pp 397–398.)* Morning stiffness that improves as the day progresses is frequently seen in ankylosing spondylitis. Psoriatic arthropathy is usually associated with the silvery cutaneous plaques that are the hallmark of psoriasis. The "sicca complex" of dry mouth and dry eyes is frequently encountered in patients with Sjögren's syndrome, while the butterfly rash is one of the eleven criteria upon which a diagnosis of systemic lupus erythematosus may be made.

28–31. The answers are 28-A, 29-E, 30-B, 31-C. *(Isselbacher, 13/e, pp 369–371, 2041–2043.)* The patient with Down's syndrome (trisomy 21) has a characteristic facial appearance that includes epicanthal folds, broad nose, open mouth, protruding tongue, and square ears. Testicular atrophy, gynecomastia, and eunuchoid appearance are features of Klinefelter's syndrome (47,XXY). Turner's syndrome (45,X or mosaics) is typified by webbed neck, short stature, and, frequently, congenital heart defects. Edwards' syndrome (trisomy 18) is a rare, sublethal condition that manifests with prominent occiput, low-set ears, micrognathia, cleft lip and palate, and flexion deformities of the fingers.

32–35. The answers are 32-D, 33-C, 34-E, 35-B. *(Isselbacher, 13/e, pp 2469–2472.)* *Latrodectus mactans* (black widow) is often found along stony walls, garages, or outhouses. The initial bite may not be felt, but symptoms of intense muscle pains, tightening about the chest, abdominal rigidity, and periodic, excruciating, cramping pains may last for 2 or 3 days. Tick paralysis caused by the hard ticks *Dermacentor andersoni* and *D. variabilis* begins as nonspecific numbness or irritability followed by weakness in the legs and an ascending flaccid paralysis; removal of the tick results in the return of normal function in hours to weeks. Human infestation with *Trombicula* larvae (chiggers) is most commonly seen as extremely pruritic, papular or papulourticarial lesions located along straps and bands of clothing with persistent burning and itching up to weeks. *Loxosceles reclusa* bites can produce the serious condition of necrotic arachnidism. The lesion becomes cyanotic with central necrosis, and the resultant ulcer may persist for weeks to months. The pajaroello tick produces painful, hemorrhagic lesions.

36–39. The answers are 36-C, 37-B, 38-A, 39-E. *(Isselbacher, 13/e, pp 226–232, 282, 299, 1468, 1970–1972.)* A Caucasian patient who appears to have a perpetual tan should be evaluated for Addison's disease, often associated with hypersecretion of melanin along with ACTH. Yellow skin with yellow sclerae is typical of jaundice, which may be secondary to viral hepatitis. Acquired blue-gray skin with dark maculae and hyperkeratosis of the palms and soles may be seen in cases of chronic arsenic ingestion. Green-yellow skin may be secondary to quinacrine therapy.

40–43. The answers are 40-A, 41-B, 42-D, 43-C. *(Isselbacher, 13/e, pp 102–104, 2088–2095.)* Arcus senilis is a degenerative change in the cornea normally seen in adults over 60 years of age. A gray band of corneal opacity in a patient under 40 years of age frequently signals hyperlipidemia. The Kayser-Fleischer ring is a band of golden-brown pigment on the posterior corneal surface; it is characteristic of hepatolenticular degeneration (Wilson's disease). Chalazions are granulomatous inflammations of the meibomian gland. A pterygium is a vascular, membranous growth across the cornea whose development is thought to be stimulated by wind and dust. Pterygia are usually horizontal and frequently bilateral growths.

44–50. The answers are 44-A; 45-B; 46-G; 47-H; 48-F; 49-E, F; 50-D. *(Isselbacher, 13/e, pp 203, 297, 778–790, 1366–1372, 1520–1532, 1940–1941, 2024, 2270–2278.)* Both acute pancreatitis and perforated ulcer frequently present with severe abdominal pain that generally starts in the upper abdomen. In both disorders the pain may radiate to the back. Rebound pain and abdominal guarding are frequent findings in a perforated ulcer. Patients with pancreatitis often present leaning forward in a chair to minimize the pain. While vomiting is frequently associated with pancreatitis, it provides very little relief. Periorbital edema is one of the classic findings in hypothyroidism as well as in nephrotic syndrome. Thus, a history of renal problems or the presence of coarse hair or other findings of myxedema may help in making the correct diagnosis. Stooped posture, resting tremor, and festinating (shuffling) gait are characteristic signs exhibited by parkinsonian patients. Neuroleptic medications may produce extrapyramidal symptoms that are indistinguishable from Parkinson's disease but are reversible when the medication is discontinued. Both Parkinson's and Alzheimer's diseases present most commonly in the elderly. While dementia is perhaps the most prominent feature of Alzheimer's disease, it is also observed in a sizable percentage of patients with Parkinson's disease. Measles generally presents with a pro-drome of fever, malaise, headache, and myalgia, followed closely by the development of photophobia and burning eye pain. White spots on the buccal mucosa (Koplik's spots) may develop during this prodromal phase. Two to four days later, the characteristic maculopapular rash appears first on the face and neck, then subsequently spreads across the trunk and to the extremities. A demyelinating encephalomyelitis is a rare but serious complication of measles and carries a 10 percent mortality. A recent study suggests that treatment of children with measles with supplemental vitamin A may reduce the incidence of major complications and death. The rash of chickenpox has a centripetal distribution and can be recognized readily by the characteristic vesicles with erythematous bases. The neurologic complications of chickenpox include encephalitis, optic neuritis, and Guillain-Barré syndrome.

Head, Eyes, Ears, Nose, and Throat

DIRECTIONS: Each item below contains a question or incomplete statement followed by suggested responses. Select the **one best** response to each question.

51. All the following are signs of complete airway obstruction EXCEPT

(A) clutching the neck with thumb and fingers
(B) inability to speak
(C) inability to cough
(D) inability to breathe
(E) high-pitched noise with inhalation

52. A normal tympanic membrane contains all the following EXCEPT

(A) pearly gray tympanic membrane
(B) light reflex (cone of light)
(C) umbo
(D) dense white plaques on the tympanic membrane
(E) chordae tympani

53. A Rinne test detects what kind of deafness?

(A) Conduction
(B) Sensorineural
(C) Electrical
(D) Hysterical
(E) None of the above

54. A patient with decreased visual acuity as determined by a Snellen chart should have which of the following tests done to rule out refraction error?

(A) Slit-lamp examination
(B) Pinhole test
(C) Pseudochromatic plate test
(D) Schiotz tonometry
(E) Visual field examination

55. A white reflex on examination of the optic fundus of an infant is most suggestive of

(A) retinoblastoma
(B) malignant melanoma
(C) retinocerebellar angioma
(D) choroidal angioma
(E) primary congenital glaucoma

56. A pituitary tumor will usually cause what kind of visual field defect?

(A) Bitemporal hemianopsia
(B) Left homonymous hemianopsia
(C) Right homonymous hemianopsia
(D) Right homonymous inferior quadrantanopia
(E) Left homonymous inferior quadrantanopia

57. A 45-year-old man presents to your office with a pituitary tumor that produces an excess amount of growth hormone. You would expect to find all the following physical findings EXCEPT

(A) a prominent brow and jaw
(B) enlargement of the lip, ears, and nose
(C) large hands
(D) exophthalmos
(E) coarse facial features

58. A 5-year-old boy presents to your office complaining of right ear pain. Upon examination of the ear, pain is elicited with traction of the tragus, the tympanic membrane is not visualized well, and some peri-auricular lymph nodes are palpable. The most likely diagnosis is

(A) acute otitis media
(B) acute otitis externa
(C) mastoiditis
(D) a blocked eustachian tube
(E) acute viral conjunctivitis

59. Hypertrophied gums are the result of which of the following?

(A) Vitamin B_{12} deficiency
(B) Administration of tetracycline
(C) Administration of diphenyl-hydantoin (phenytoin)
(D) Fluoride overdose
(E) Vitamin D-resistant rickets

60. Which of the following can cause a discoloration of the lips seen on physical examination?

(A) Congenital syphilis
(B) Neurofibromatosis
(C) Peutz-Jeghers syndrome
(D) Familial polyposis
(E) Rheumatic fever

61. Hyperthyroidism is caused by an excess amount of thyroid hormone. All the following would be expected on physical examination EXCEPT

(A) fine, oily hair
(B) ocular muscle paresis
(C) tremor
(D) a thyroid bruit
(E) bradycardia

62. All the following are characteristics of Horner's syndrome EXCEPT

(A) miosis
(B) enophthalmos
(C) ptosis
(D) facial palsy
(E) anhidrosis of the ipsilateral side of the face

63. According to the cardinal positions of gaze, which of the following pairings of ocular muscles and actions is correct?

(A) Inferior oblique muscle—abduction and elevation
(B) Lateral rectus muscle—adduction
(C) Medial rectus muscle—abduction and depression
(D) Superior oblique muscle—adduction and depression
(E) Superior rectus muscle—depression

64. A 66-year-old patient presents to you with a complaint of a swelling in the neck. Upon examination you note a 2-cm hard, firm nodule in the posterior triangle of the left side of the neck. Which of the following would you do next?

(A) Examine the lung fields
(B) Examine the oral cavity
(C) Perform a Weber test
(D) Perform a visual acuity test
(E) Reassure the patient that the mass will go away

65. A 58-year-old man presents to your office with a history of having an episode of sudden visual loss in his right eye. The patient describes the loss of vision as similar to someone pulling a cover over his right eye. Vision returned to the right eye after 10 min. This visual field defect is

(A) scotoma
(B) amaurosis fugax
(C) strabismus
(D) esotropia
(E) night blindness

66. Funduscopic examination of a patient with transient ischemic attacks (TIA) may reveal what physical finding?

(A) Hollenhorst plaques
(B) Papilledema
(C) Cotton-wool spots
(D) AV nicking
(E) Capillary aneurysms

67. A positive Chvostek's sign is seen in which of the following conditions?

(A) Hypokalemia
(B) Hypercalcemia
(C) Hypocalcemia
(D) Hyperkalemia
(E) Hypernatremia

68. A young man presents to your office after suffering blunt trauma to his right eye. Examination of the eye reveals normal pupillary response, but blood in the anterior chamber. This condition is called

(A) external hordeolum
(B) internal hordeolum
(C) chalazion
(D) hyphema
(E) cataract

69. A young man presents with a history of right facial pain, headache, and stuffy nose. Upon examination you find swollen, pale nasal mucosa, tenderness over the right maxillary sinus, and a right maxillary sinus that does not transilluminate. The most probable diagnosis is

(A) mononucleosis
(B) acute streptococcal pharyngitis
(C) acute sinusitis
(D) tension headache
(E) acute glaucoma

70. Breath with a fruity smell is most characteristic of

(A) diabetes mellitus
(B) fetor hepaticus
(C) oral candidiasis
(D) lung abscess
(E) uremia

71. All the following are associated with occlusion of the retinal vein EXCEPT

(A) slow, progressive, unilateral loss of vision
(B) retinal and macular edema
(C) loss of lateral gaze
(D) arteriosclerosis
(E) cotton-wool patches

72. The best test to determine if there is corneal abrasion is

(A) tonometry
(B) fluorescein stain
(C) pinhole test
(D) funduscopy
(E) visual field test

73. When performing a Weber test, there is lateralization to the right ear. A Rinne test shows that bone conduction is greater than air conduction. What type of hearing loss does this describe?

(A) Sensorineural hearing loss on the right
(B) Sensorineural hearing loss on the left
(C) Bilateral conduction deafness
(D) Conduction deafness on the left
(E) Normal bilateral hearing

74. Which of the following is the best method to palpate the thyroid gland?

(A) From behind the patient
(B) Using the palms of your hands
(C) While the patient is talking
(D) Starting with the chin and working down
(E) With the patient's chin on his or her chest

75. A 6-year-old boy presents to your office with a history of neck stiffness following an upper respiratory infection. On examination you note that the patient's head is leaning toward the left shoulder and slightly rotated. The most likely diagnosis is

(A) acute meningitis
(B) thoracic spinal deformity
(C) torticollis
(D) scoliosis
(E) goiter

76. A 60-year-old man presents with a small lesion on his nose. On examination of the lesion you note that the lesion is 3 mm in diameter and is slightly elevated with a waxy appearance and a slight vascular pattern on top. This lesion is most characteristic of which of the following?

(A) Basal cell carcinoma
(B) Squamous cell carcinoma
(C) Melanoma
(D) Aphthous ulcer
(E) Bowen's disease

77. Examination of a patient's visual field reveals complete blindness in the left eye. Ophthalmoscopic examination is normal. At what level is the lesion?

(A) Between the optic chiasma and the lateral geniculate body
(B) Between the retina and the optic chiasma
(C) Between the lateral geniculate body and the visual cortex
(D) At the medial longitudinal fasciculus
(E) At the visual cortex

78. When testing a patient's extraocular muscle movements, you note that the right eye cannot adduct past the midline. However, when you move a fingertip toward the patient's nose, convergence does occur. This condition is

(A) paralysis of cranial nerve VI
(B) paralysis of cranial nerve III
(C) internuclear ophthalmoplegia
(D) Bell's palsy
(E) retrobulbar optic neuritis

79. A patient complains of unilateral headache and tenderness of the right temple. Inspection reveals a slightly swollen right temple. Palpation reveals an enlarged, tender right temporal artery. The most likely diagnosis is

(A) acute frontal sinusitis
(B) acute maxillary sinusitis
(C) giant cell arteritis
(D) cluster headache
(E) migraine headache

80. A 4-year-old presents with sudden onset of sore throat, hoarseness, and difficulty breathing. The patient prefers to lean forward, is drooling, and has a high temperature. The most likely diagnosis is

(A) acute epiglottitis
(B) whooping cough
(C) streptococcal pharyngitis
(D) bronchiolitis
(E) mononucleosis

81. A thyroid bruit is associated with which of the following?

(A) A thyroductal cyst
(B) Ectopic thyroid
(C) Thyroiditis
(D) Graves' disease
(E) Thyroid goiter

82. A unilateral neck mass could be any of the following EXCEPT

(A) a thyroductal cyst
(B) a brachial cleft cyst
(C) a lipoma
(D) a carotid body tumor
(E) an enlarged cervical lymph node

83. A tracheal tug, or Oliver's sign, is seen in which of the following conditions?

(A) Aortic aneurysm
(B) Thyroid goiter
(C) Carotid body tumor
(D) Lipoma
(E) Thyroductal cyst

84. When a patient presents with hoarseness, the differential diagnosis should include all the following EXCEPT

(A) Pancoast's tumor
(B) vocal cord tumor
(C) laryngeal trauma
(D) goiter
(E) otitis externa

85. On physical examination, Bell's palsy is characterized by all the following EXCEPT

(A) drooping of the corner of the mouth
(B) difficulty speaking
(C) inability to close the eye on the ipsilateral side
(D) inability to abduct the ipsilateral eye
(E) drooling

86. A 51-year-old indigent man presents to the emergency room with horizontal nystagmus, ataxic gait, and confusion. Which of the following is the most likely diagnosis?

(A) Middle cerebral artery infarct
(B) Thiamine deficiency
(C) Niacin deficiency
(D) Viral encephalitis .
(E) Pellagra

87. A 46-year-old woman presents with drooping eyelids, but no other significant findings. Which of the following diagnoses should be considered?

(A) Bell's palsy
(B) Metastatic tumor impinging upon the cervical sympathetic trunk
(C) Hyperthyroidism
(D) Myasthenia gravis
(E) Reiter's syndrome

DIRECTIONS: Each group of questions below consists of lettered options followed by numbered items. For each numbered item, select the appropriate lettered option(s). Each lettered option may be used once, more than once, or not at all. **Choose exactly the number of options indicated following each item.**

Items 88–91

Match each ocular condition with its cause.

(A) Abnormal copper deposition
(B) Abnormal triangular fold of membrane extending from the conjunctiva to the cornea
(C) Conjunctival edema
(D) Acute purulent infection of the meibomian gland of the eyelid
(E) Yellow-white discoloration around the periphery of the cornea

88. Hordeolum **(SELECT 1 CAUSE)**

89. Arcus senilis **(SELECT 1 CAUSE)**

90. Pterygium **(SELECT 1 CAUSE)**

91. Kayser-Fleischer rings **(SELECT 1 CAUSE)**

Items 92–95

For each of the clinical conditions below, match the test most appropriate.

(A) Tonometry
(B) Transillumination
(C) Pinhole test
(D) Cover test
(E) Chvostek's test (sign)

92. Strabismus **(SELECT 1 TEST)**

93. Refractory errors **(SELECT 1 TEST)**

94. Sinusitis **(SELECT 1 TEST)**

95. Glaucoma **(SELECT 1 TEST)**

DIRECTIONS: Each group of questions below consists of four lettered options followed by a set of numbered items. For each numbered item select

A	if the item is associated with	(A) only
B	if the item is associated with	(B) only
C	if the item is associated with	**both** (A) and (B)
D	if the item is associated with	**neither** (A) nor (B)

Each lettered option may be used **once, more than once, or not at all.**

Items 96–98

  (A) Argyll Robertson pupil
  (B) Adie's tonic pupil
  (C) Both
  (D) Neither

96. Accommodation

97. Response to direct light stimulation

98. Bilateralness

Items 99–101

  (A) Aphthous stomatitis
  (B) Herpetic gingivostomatitis
  (C) Both
  (D) Neither

99. Painless ulcer

100. Primary vesicular lesions

101. Occurrence in clusters

Items 102–105

  (A) Facial nerve (cranial nerve VII)
  (B) Trigeminal nerve (cranial nerve V)
  (C) Both
  (D) Neither

102. Facial expression

103. Pupillary reflex

104. Muscles of mastication

105. Corneal reflex

Items 106–108

  (A) Allergic rhinitis
  (B) Viral rhinitis
  (C) Both
  (D) Neither

106. Reddened nasal mucosa

107. Eosinophils on nasal smear

108. Pale, boggy nasal mucosa

Items 109–111

    (A) Leukoplakia
    (B) Thrush (oral candidiasis)
    (C) Both
    (D) Neither

109. Patchy, white oral lesions

110. Premalignant lesions

111. Treatment with oral antibiotics

Items 112–115

    (A) Acute bacterial
         conjunctivitis
    (B) Allergic (atopic)
         conjunctivitis
    (C) Both
    (D) Neither

112. Purulent discharge

113. Severe itching

114. Ciliary flush

115. Preauricular adenopathy

Head, Eyes, Ears, Nose, and Throat

Answers

51. The answer is E. *(Emergency Cardiac Care Committee, JAMA 268:2174, 1992.)* Signs of complete airway obstruction include clutching the neck with thumb and fingers (universal distress signal) and inability to speak, breathe, or cough. With a complete obstruction, there is no air exchange, and therefore patients generally will make no sounds with attempted breathing. A partial obstruction may cause a weak, ineffective cough; high-pitched noise with inhalation; and respiratory difficulty.

52. The answer is D. *(Sapira, pp 209–211.)* The normal tympanic membrane is pinkish-to-pearly gray in color and has a light reflex. The umbo is in the lower portion of the malleus. Occasionally the chordae tympani can be seen traversing the tympanic membrane. Dense white plaques may be tympanosclerosis.

53. The answer is A. *(Sapira, pp 211–213.)* The Rinne test is performed by placing a tuning fork (512 Hz) over the mastoid process. When vibration is no longer heard by bone conduction, the tuning fork is placed near the ear to determine if vibration is heard. If the vibration is heard, then air conduction is greater than bone conduction and the test is considered positive, or normal. However, if the vibration is not heard, then bone conduction is greater than air conduction and this negative Rinne test denotes conduction deafness.

54. The answer is B. *(Delp, 9/e, p 165. Vaughan, 13/e, pp 21–54.)* A pinhole test allows only paraxial parallel light rays through and improves visual acuity if refractory errors are present. The slit-lamp examination is a direct visualization of the eye and its components. The pseudochromatic plate test detects color blindness. Schiotz tonometry measures intraocular pressure. Visual field testing determines if there are any blind spots.

55. The answer is A. *(Hathaway, 11/e, pp 376, 404, 415–416, 717–718.)* Malignant melanoma is the most common tumor but must be differentiated from a benign nevus. Retinoblastoma is a malignant tumor that is seen rarely in infants and children and causes a white reflex. Retinocerebellar angiomatosis, von Hippel-Lindau disease, is a rare, dominantly inherited disease in which the patient may present with ataxia, slurred speech, nystagmus, and retinal detachment. Diagnosis is made with findings of retinal or cerebellar hemangioblastoma and an intraabdominal cyst or renal cancer. Choroidal angioma is found in Sturge-Weber disease. The eye finding is congenital glaucoma or buphthalmos (marked enlargement of the eye at birth) with an enlarged, cloudy cornea. Primary congenital glaucoma is a condition of increased intraocular pressure caused by abnormal development of aqueous drainage structures.

56. The answer is A. *(Delp, 9/e, pp 96-97. Vaughan, 13/e, pp 234–235.)* A pituitary tumor may impinge on the optic chiasm. The temporal field fibers are damaged as they decussate at the optic chiasm and the result is a bitemporal hemianopsia. The nasal field fibers do not cross and are spared early in the disease process.

57. The answer is D. *(Delp, 9/e, pp 142–144.)* The increased release of growth hormone causes an increase in growth of both soft tissue and bone. Therefore, you would see an increase in hand size, a prominent brow and jaw, plus an increase in the soft tissues of the lips, ears, and nose. Exophthalmos is associated with increased levels of thyroid hormone.

58. The answer is B. *(Hathaway, 11/e, pp 440–441.)* Acute otitis externa is the infection of the external auditory canal. The external canal can swell, which makes examination of the tympanic membrane difficult. Pulling on the tragus, or the pinna, extends the canal and causes pain. Palpable lymphadenopathy involving the periauricular and cervical lymph nodes may be present. Debris is often seen in the canal and the patient resists all attempts at speculum examination.

59. The answer is C. *(Isselbacher, 13/e, pp 410, 604.)* Use of the anticonvulsant diphenylhydantoin or of the antianginal calcium channel blocker nifedipine may cause fibrous hyperplasia of the gingiva, or hypertrophied gums. It is an unsightly covering of the teeth that may interfere with eating. Tetracycline given in the latter half of pregnancy or up until 8 years of age may cause enamel hypoplasia and discoloration of the teeth. Daily ingestion of more than 1.5 mg of fluoride can cause mottling of the tooth enamel. Vitamin D-resistant rickets causes enamel hypoplasia that ranges from white spots to gross structural changes of the teeth.

60. The answer is C. *(Isselbacher, 13/e, pp 297, 1425, 2024, 2339.)* Peutz-Jeghers syndrome is a familial disorder that includes hamartomas of the colon and pigmented lesions of the lips and buccal mucosa. Congenital syphilis and rheumatic fever cause a generalized systemic rash of the skin. Familial polyposis is a disorder characterized by colonic polyps. Neurofibromatosis has characteristic cream-brown cutaneous lesions (café-au-lait spots).

61. The answer is E. *(Isselbacher, 13/e, 1941–1948.).* Hyperthyroidism is an overproduction of thyroid hormone that causes fine, oily hair, a variety of extraocular muscle palsies, tremor, weight loss, and a thyroid bruit from the increased vascularization of the thyroid. Increased thyroid hormone causes a tachycardia.

62. The answer is D. *(Isselbacher, 13/e, pp 102, 149, 2344, 2351.)* Horner's syndrome is caused by the loss of sympathetic innervation to one side of the face and neck. With loss of this innervation, the pupil becomes constricted, the eyelid droops, the eye is somewhat sunken, and there is loss of sweating on the ipsilateral side of sympathetic loss. Loss of innervation by cranial nerve VII causes ipsilateral facial muscle paralysis, or facial palsy.

63. The answer is D. *(Moore, 3/e, p 716–717.)* According to the cardinal positions of gaze, the medial rectus muscle adducts, the lateral rectus muscle abducts, the superior rectus muscle elevates, the inferior rectus muscle depresses, the inferior oblique muscle adducts and elevates, and the superior oblique muscle adducts and depresses.

64. The answer is B. *(Delp, 9/e, pp 137–139.)* Firm, hard, nontender lymph nodes in the neck are often due to distant malignancy. The oral cavity should be examined very carefully for a primary malignancy. Patients with malignancy of the face, lips, oral cavity, and larynx may present with enlarged lymph nodes. Other sources of malignancy are the thyroid, which involves the anterior cervical lymph nodes, and lymphomas, chest malignancies, and abdominal malignancies, which may involve the supraclavicular nodes (Virchow's nodes).

65. The answer is B. *(Isselbacher, 13/e, pp 2204, 2234.)* The patient is describing a transient ischemic attack (TIA). These attacks occur suddenly and produce reversible, unilateral visual loss or neurologic deficits. The attacks last from a few minutes to a few hours. These attacks are produced by emboli that occlude the retinal artery and may be associated with carotid atherosclerosis, which may be the source of emboli. Auscultation of the carotids may reveal a bruit.

66. The answer is A. *(Seidel, 3/e, pp 249–254, 263–268.)* On examination of the fundus, you may see Hollenhorst plaques. These are cholesterol emboli that are lodged in the retinal artery. They arise from an atheromatous plaque and contain both cholesterol and fibrin. These emboli originate from plaques in the carotid arteries, and auscultation of the carotid arteries may reveal bruits. The other funduscopic findings are seen in both hypertensive and diabetic retinopathy.

67. The answer is C. *(Talley, 2/e, p 296.)* A Chvostek's sign is elicited by tapping on cranial nerve VII as it exits the parotid gland. In states of hypocalcemia (tetany), a positive test shows spasm or contraction of facial muscles on the same side as the nerve that is being tapped. This finding is pathognomonic for tetany, which may be secondary to hypoparathyroidism.

68. The answer is D. *(Hathaway, 11/e, pp 405–406. Vaughan, 13/e, pp 347, 426–429.)* A common sequela of blunt trauma to the eye is a hyphema (blood in the anterior chamber). This is caused by rupture of small blood vessels lying close to the cornea. Chalazion is a granulomatous infection of the meibomian glands that causes a slight discomfort and redness to the eyelid with a small lump on the palpebral surface. An external hordeolum is an abscess of the sebaceous glands on the lid margin; an internal hordeolum is an infection of the meibomian glands that usually appears on the conjunctival surface of the lid. A cataract is opacity of the lens caused by precipitated lens proteins.

69. The answer is C. *(Isselbacher, 13/e, pp 516–517. Hathaway, 11/e, pp 450–452.)* This is a classic history of someone presenting with acute maxillary sinusitis. When a sinus becomes swollen and inflamed, facial pain can be elicited by percussing over the involved sinus. The patient may also have headache, fever, postnasal drip, or purulent rhinorrhea. In a darkened room, hold a thin beam of bright light against the maxillary sinus and attempt to observe light in the oral cavity. Asymmetry suggests that the nontransilluminating sinus is filled with purulent material.

70. The answer is A. *(Delp, 9/e, p 156. Sapira, pp 228–229.)* In a diabetic patient in ketosis, acetone is excreted in the lungs and gives the breath a fruity smell. The patient with liver disease has a musty smell, or *fetor hepaticus*. A patient with uremia has breath that smells of ammonia. Patients with lung abscess have a very putrid breath odor called *fetor oris*.

71. The answer is C. *(Isselbacher, 13/e, p 104.)* Occlusion of the retinal vein occurs from slow venous blood flow and thrombosis. The patient usually presents with progressive unilateral loss of vision. On funduscopy, you can see retinal and macular edema, tortuous veins, and retinal hemorrhages with an occasional cotton-wool patch. The funduscopic image is so dramatic that the description "blood and thunder" is often used.

72. The answer is B. *(Seidel, 3/e, pp 242–266.)* Abrasions of the cornea can be visualized under cobalt blue lighting after the instillation of fluorescein stain. Vertical scratches (defects) are nearly pathognomonic for foreign bodies under the upper eyelid. Tonometry only measures intraocular pressure. Funduscopy is done to visualize the optic disc, retinal blood vessels, retinal background, and macula. If there is improvement in visual acuity when the patient reads through a pinhole, then the visual disturbance is most likely a refractive error, most commonly myopia, which becomes symptomatic in school-aged children.

73. The answer is A. *(Sapira, pp 211–213.)* A Weber test is performed by placing the tuning fork against the top of the head in the midline. If the sound is heard in both ears equally, then it is a normal test. If the sound is heard better in one ear than the other, it lateralizes to the side of neural deafness. The Rinne test determines if air conduction is greater than bone conduction. If bone conduction is greater than air conduction, then there is sensorineural damage. The Weber and Rinne tests complement each other.

74. The answer is A. *(Sapira, pp 231–233.)* To palpate the thyroid gland effectively, have the patient sit down in a comfortable position. Then from behind the patient, palpate the thyroid cartilage and move down until you feel the cricoid cartilage. This is the area of the isthmus of the thyroid. Now carefully move laterally, palpating with your fingertips. Have the patient swallow and feel the thyroid gland move up and down.

75. The answer is C. *(Hathaway, 11/e, p 751.)* The most likely diagnosis is torticollis. This is a condition in which the sternomastoid muscle is shortened by muscle spasm or fibrosis. The shortening of the sternomastoid muscle pulls the head down toward the affected side and causes rotation of the head to the opposite side of the involved muscle.

76. The answer is A. *(Isselbacher, 13/e, pp A2–A20, 272, 309, 1866.)* Basal cell carcinomas of the face are found primarily above the level of the mouth. These lesions are slow-growing and waxy with a vascular pattern on the surface. They may eventually ulcerate in the middle and produce the "rat bite ulcer." Squamous cell carcinomas (SCC) commonly occur in sun-damaged skin or chronic lesions and tend to have a noduloulcerative appearance with rolled-up margins. Melanomas are associated with heavy exposure to the sun and are multiple colors. Aphthous ulcers are lesions of the oral pharynx. Bowen's disease is the most prevalent form of SCC in situ and may mimic chronic eczema, though SCC is quite erythematous with very sharp borders.

77. The answer is B. *(Isselbacher, 13/e, pp 104–106, 2321–2348. Seidel, 3/e, p 267.)* When defects are detected in only one eye, the lesion is anterior to the optic chiasma. Lesions at the optic chiasma produce bitemporal hemianopia because this is where nasal retinal fibers decussate. The medial longitudinal fasciculus is involved with extraocular muscle coordination. Lesions between the geniculate body and visual cortex would produce a contralateral upper homonymous quadrantanopia. Because fibers subserving similar areas of the retinas become very close as they travel posteriorly to the occipital lobes (visual cortex), a lesion in the visual cortex would produce similar field defects in each eye.

78. The answer is C. *(Isselbacher, 13/e, pp 108, 2289.)* Internuclear ophthalmoplegia (INO) is due to a lesion in the medial longitudinal fasciculus (MLF). It is usually caused by a glioma in children, multiple sclerosis in young adults, or vascular infarction in the geriatric population. INO commonly consists of paresis of adduction of the ipsilateral eye, horizontal jerk nystagmus in the contralateral abducting eye, intact convergence, and vertical nystagmus with upward gaze.

79. The answer is C. *(Isselbacher, 13/e, pp 204, 1676–1677.)* Giant cell (temporal) arteritis usually appears after age 55 and is more common in women. Patients typically present with headache, malaise, fever, tenderness over the involved artery, and polymyalgia rheumatica (limb-girdle pain) and eventually may have ocular symptoms secondary to ischemic optic neuropathy. They may complain of pain when combing their hair. Jaw pain when chewing (jaw claudication) is nearly pathognomonic.

80. The answer is A. *(Isselbacher, 13/e, pp 519, 618–619.)* The epiglottis is markedly swollen, cherry-red, and sensitive, such that stimulation of the posterior oral pharynx could precipitate laryngeal spasm and obstruction. Therefore, the diagnosis is made primarily on history and lateral x-rays of the soft tissue of the neck. Other complaints are dysphagia, odynophagia, and fever that has rapidly progressed. Hoarseness and loss of voice power are universal findings. Stridor may be present. The difference between acute epiglottitis and streptococcal pharyngitis is that the onset of streptococcal pharyngitis is slower (days versus hours).

81. The answer is D. *(Delp, 9/e, p 135. Sapira, p 234.)* A bruit is turbulent blood flow heard with a stethoscope. In Graves' disease, there is a hypervascular gland with increased blood flow. The bruit is almost pathognomonic for Graves' disease. It is best heard over the lateral lobes. One must be careful not to mistake a cardiac murmur transmitted through the carotid artery for a thyroid bruit.

82. The answer is A. *(Delp, 9/e, pp 133–141.)* All the listed entities except a thyroductal cyst are lateral to the midline of the neck. A thyroductal cyst, a midline structure, is a remnant of the passage of the thyroid from the base of the tongue into the neck. A lipoma is a fatty tumor that can be found anywhere in the subcutaneous tissue. The neck has several groups of lymph nodes, any of which may be enlarged. A carotid body tumor arises from the carotid body located at the bifurcation of the common carotid artery.

83. The answer is A. *(Delp, 9/e, p 141. Sapira, p 235.)* A tracheal tug was described by William Silver Oliver, an English physician. The sign is elicited when the patient sits erect, mouth closed, chin extended, and the trachea pulled upward by the examiner. If an aortic aneurysm is present, the pulsations may be transmitted through the trachea to the examiner's hand. The aorta arches over the left main stem bronchus, and when the trachea is stretched, the dilated aorta pulsates against the bronchus, thus transmitting the pulses upward.

84. The answer is E. *(Delp, 9/e, p 160.)* Hoarseness is due to edema or swelling of the larynx or vocal cords, or to external compression of the larynx or recurrent laryngeal nerve. Pancoast's tumor of the thorax may cause recurrent laryngeal nerve compression. Laryngeal trauma causes swelling and inflammation. Vocal cord tumors, often associated with heavy smoking, cause decreased flexibility of the vocal cords. Otitis externa is an infection of the external ear canal that does not cause hoarseness.

85. The answer is D. *(Delp, 9/e, p 108. Sapira, pp 458–459.)* Bell's palsy is the loss of motor function of cranial nerve VII to the ipsilateral side of the face. This causes drooping of the mouth and facial muscles, inability to close the ipsilateral eye, and difficulty speaking and eating. With the drooping of the mouth, the patient may have trouble with drooling from the corner of the mouth on the affected side. Abduction of the eye is controlled by cranial nerve VI.

86. The answer is B. *(Isselbacher, 13/e, pp 474, 2421.)* The triad of nystagmus, ataxia, and confusion is associated with the Wernicke-Korsakoff syndrome, often seen in poorly nourished alcoholics. While strokes and encephalitides may present with a confusional state and motor dysfunction, they would be less likely than thiamine deficiency in an indigent patient.

Niacin deficiency (pellagra) classically presents with the triad of dermatitis, diarrhea, and dementia.

87.   The answer is D. *(Isselbacher, 13/e, pp 102, 145, 761, 764, 1942–1946, 2344, 2349–2350.)* A unilateral ptosis is associated with Horner's syndrome, which is caused by interruption of the cervical sympathetic chain. Bilateral drooping of the eyelids may be an early sign of myasthenia gravis. Bell's palsy and hyperthyroidism both tend to cause lid retraction and a staring gaze. Conjunctivitis constitutes part of the classic triad of Reiter's syndrome.

88–91.   The answers are 88-D, 89-E, 90-B, 91-A. *(Delp, 9/e, pp 174–175. Sapira, p 165. Vaughan, 13/e, pp 426–429.)* A hordeolum is an acute infection of the meibomian gland and is usually caused by staphylococci. Arcus senilis is a benign condition in the elderly due to deposition of lipids around the cornea. If seen in a younger person, it may be a marker for hyperlipidemia. A pterygium is an abnormal triangular fold of membrane that extends from the conjunctiva to the cornea; it is due to irritation by ultraviolet light, dust, or sand. Kayser-Fleischer rings are seen in persons with Wilson's disease. They have abnormal copper metabolism and deposit copper into body tissues, which is observable in the eye.

92–95.   The answers are 92-D, 93-C, 94-B, 95-A. *(Delp, 9/e, pp 163–166. Vaughan, 13/e, pp 26–27, 713.)* The cover test removes fixation of one eye and allows the other eye to come to fixation for the purpose of noting strabismus. Transillumination of the sinuses can aid in diagnosing sinusitis by the presence of opacification. Tonometry measures the elevated intraocular pressure of glaucoma. People who have subnormal vision secondary to refractory errors will have improvement in visual acuity with the pinhole test. Chvostek's sign is elicited by tapping on the facial nerve where it exits the parotid gland. The positive response that is seen in hypocalcemia is tetanic spasms of the ipsilateral muscles of facial expression.

96–98.   The answers are 96-A, 97-D, 98-A. *(Delp, 9/e, pp 99, 170. Vaughan, 13/e, pp 261–262. Sapira, pp 170–173.)* Argyll Robertson pupil is usually miotic (<3 mm) and almost always bilateral. The pupil does not react to direct light stimulation but will react to accommodation. An Argyll Robertson pupil is suggestive of neurosyphilis that affects the light reflex pathway. An Adie's tonic pupil is a dysfunction of the constrictor muscle; therefore, it does not respond to direct light or to accommodation.

99–101.   The answers are 99-D, 100-B, 101-C. *(Delp, 9/e, p 159. Sapira, p 226.)* Aphthous ulcers are painful oral ulcers located on the buccal mucosa and gingiva. They are a grayish lesion on a red base and never start as vesicular lesions. Herpetic gingivostomatitis is a herpetic lesion usually found on the vermilion border, but it can also affect the buccal mucosa and gingiva. These lesions start as vesicles and then ulcerate. They are painful and regress with time.

102–105. The answers are 102-A, 103-D, 104-B, 105-C. *(Delp, 9/e, pp 95–104. Sapira, pp 457–458.)* Cranial nerve V has both sensory and motor functions. It supplies sensation to the face and motion to the muscles of mastication. It also provides the afferent fibers for the corneal reflex. Cranial nerve VII supplies the muscles of facial expression, including muscles responsible for the blink of the corneal reflex. Cranial nerve III supplies motion to almost all the extraocular muscles and the efferent fibers of the pupillary reflex.

106–108. The answers are 106-B, 107-A, 108-A. *(Hathaway, 11/e, pp 446–449, 956–958.)* Viral rhinitis produces a reddened, moist nasal mucosa, which suggests irritation. Allergic rhinitis produces a pale, boggy mucosa secondary to edema and swelling. Eosinophils on a nasal smear colored by Giemsa stain are suggestive of an allergic reaction.

109–111. The answers are 109-C, 110-A, 111-D. *(Delp, 9/e, pp 157–159. Sapira, p 223.)* Both leukoplakia and thrush appear as white, patchy lesions of the oral mucosa. Thrush is easily scraped off, whereas leukoplakia is not. Leukoplakia results from chronic irritation and is prone to become malignant. It is treated by removal of the irritating agent or by surgical means. Thrush, which is secondary to a *Candida* infection, is treated with an antifungal agent.

112–115. The answers are 112-A, 113-B, 114-D, 115-D. *(Delp, 9/e, pp 178–179. Sapira, p 166. Vaughan, 13/e, pp 74–82, 84–87.)* A purulent discharge is suggestive of a bacterial infection. A Gram stain of the discharge will show an increase in the white blood cells along with many bacteria.

Itching can be associated with many forms of conjunctivitis, but is most severe with allergic (atopic) conjunctivitis.

Ciliary flush is the engorgement of the deep pericorneal blood vessels. It is associated with conditions such as iridocyclitis, endophthalmitis, and glaucoma, but not superficial infections.

Preauricular adenopathy is an important physical finding. It is not seen in acute bacterial conjunctivitis or allergic (atopic) conjunctivitis, but is very common with epidemic keratoconjunctivitis (caused by adenovirus) and herpes simplex viral conjunctivitis.

Cardiovascular System

DIRECTIONS: Each item below contains a question or incomplete statement followed by suggested responses. Select the **one best** response to each question.

116. A split S_1 is most commonly caused by

(A) inspiration
(B) expiration
(C) atrial septal defect
(D) ventricular septal defect
(E) right bundle branch block

117. Which of the following symptoms would be LEAST likely to be present in an otherwise healthy 55-year-old man with an acute myocardial infarction?

(A) Dyspnea
(B) Nausea
(C) Confusion
(D) Diaphoresis
(E) Chest pain

118. The intensity of the first heart sound (S_1) may be increased by all the following conditions EXCEPT

(A) shortened PR interval
(B) augmented flow across the mitral valve
(C) mitral stenosis
(D) shortened diastole
(E) atrial fibrillation

119. All the following statements regarding the second heart sound (S_2) are true EXCEPT

(A) it is caused by the closure of the aortic and pulmonary valves
(B) a split S_2 may be a normal finding
(C) splitting of S_2 is increased by inspiration
(D) standing increases a split S_2
(E) a split S_2 is made up of A_2 followed by P_2

120. The third heart sound (S_3) is

(A) a high-pitched sound
(B) a normal finding in older patients
(C) heard in early systole
(D) associated with atrial dysfunction
(E) best heard at the apex of the heart

121. The fourth heart sound (S_4) is

(A)   absent in patients with atrial fibrillation

(B)   heard best at the base of the heart

(C)   heard best with the diaphragm of the stethoscope

(D)   not heard in patients with an acute myocardial infarct

(E)   always a normal finding

122. Inspiration increases the murmur of

(A)   tricuspid regurgitation

(B)   atrial septal defect

(C)   patent ductus arteriosus

(D)   mitral regurgitation

(E)   aortic stenosis

123. Cyclic variation of the heart rate is

(A)   pulsus alternans

(B)   pulsus paradoxus

(C)   pericarditis

(D)   sinus arrhythmia

(E)   cardiac tamponade

124. Which of the following statements regarding heart murmurs is true?

(A)   Murmurs are graded 0 to V

(B)   Grade III murmurs are loud

(C)   Grade V murmurs can be heard without contact of the stethoscope with the chest wall

(D)   Murmurs are audible sounds caused by turbulent blood flow

(E)   Murmurs are usually associated with a thrill

125. Coarse, scratchy sounds in both systole and diastole are auscultated throughout the precordium in a patient with chest pain. The likely diagnosis is

(A)   mitral valve prolapse

(B)   pericarditis

(C)   coarctation of the aorta

(D)   pneumonia

(E)   none of the above

126. Risk factors for atherosclerosis include all the following
EXCEPT

(A) high levels of high-density
lipoprotein (HDL)
(B) hypercholesterolemia
(C) cigarette smoking
(D) diabetes mellitus
(E) hypertension

127. A 37-year-old man presents
after 3 days of feeling weak. He
drinks alcohol daily. He had to
come in when he felt chest palpitations. He has shortness of breath and
lightheadedness with any exertion.
His pulse feels irregularly irregular.
The most likely diagnosis is

(A) sinus tachycardia
(B) sinus bradycardia
(C) ventricular premature beats
(D) atrial fibrillation
(E) ventricular fibrillation

128. Concerning varicose veins,
all the following statements are
true EXCEPT

(A) they are most commonly
located in the superficial veins
of the lower limbs
(B) they are more common in
females
(C) they are a sign of impending
heart failure
(D) complications include stasis
dermatitis and skin ulceration
(E) focal calcifications are
common

129. Which of the following sets
of signs and symptoms is most consistent with pulmonary embolism?

(A) Pleuritic chest pain, tachypnea,
tachycardia
(B) Fatigue, lethargy, confusion
(C) Epigastric pain, nausea,
vomiting
(D) Dyspnea, chest pain
(E) Diaphoresis, cyanosis, pallor

130. Which of the following
enzymes or isoenzymes is elevated
in the serum of patients 6 h after
acute myocardial infarction?

(A) Alanine transaminase (ALT,
or SGPT)
(B) Aspartate transaminase (AST,
or SGOT)
(C) Lactic dehydrogenase (LDH)
(D) Creatine phosphokinase (CPK)
(E) Hydroxybutyric dehydroge-
nase (HBD)

131. A 53-year-old man, who has
a 40-pack-year history of cigarette
smoking, presents with the complaint that he was awakened suddenly from sleep with palpitations
and shortness of breath. He was
afraid that he was having a "heart
attack" and hurried to the hospital.
The symptoms are now gone and he
claims never to have had exertional
angina. The most likely diagnosis is

(A) myocardial infarction
(B) atrial fibrillation
(C) Prinzmetal's angina
(D) stable angina
(E) pulmonary edema

132. All the following are *major* Jones criteria for the diagnosis of rheumatic fever EXCEPT

(A)   chorea
(B)   erythema marginatum
(C)   fever
(D)   carditis
(E)   subcutaneous nodules

133. The *a* wave of the venous pressure curve occurs at what point on a normal ECG tracing?

(A)   Simultaneously with the QRS complex
(B)   Just after the QRS complex
(C)   Just after the T wave
(D)   Prior to the P wave
(E)   Just after the P wave

134. The *a* wave of the jugular venous pulse (JVP) represents

(A)   right ventricular contraction
(B)   right atrial contraction
(C)   ventricular septal defect
(D)   atrial septal defect
(E)   persistent ductus arteriosus

135. All the following statements concerning hypertension are true EXCEPT

(A)   nearly 95 percent of all cases have an unknown etiology
(B)   a single elevated blood pressure is enough to establish the diagnosis
(C)   age, sex, race, weight, and smoking are all factors in the development of hypertension
(D)   patients with hypertension die prematurely
(E)   treatment has a large number of minor side effects, which reduces compliance

136. Pulmonary emboli are

(A)   usually from superficial leg veins
(B)   likely to occur after prolonged bed rest, immobilization, or a major operation
(C)   rarely fatal
(D)   decreased during pregnancy and can be treated prophylactically with estrogens
(E)   more common in children

137. In an adult with coarctation of the aorta

(A)   the femoral pulse is brisk, bounding, and simultaneous with the upper extremity pulse

(B)   blood pressure in the leg is greater than in the arm

(C)   the zone of narrowing is usually distal to the left subclavian artery

(D)   there is a decreased pulse pressure

(E)   there are no radiologic clues to the diagnosis

138. During a sustained Valsalva maneuver, all the following occur EXCEPT

(A)   a fall in cardiac output

(B)   an increase in heart rate

(C)   an increase in venous return

(D)   an increase in the murmur of hypertrophic aortic stenosis

(E)   a decrease in right-heart filling

139. A precordial thrill is correctly described by which of the following statements?

(A)   It is almost always a normal finding

(B)   It accompanies most murmurs

(C)   It is best timed by auscultation

(D)   It is a palpable organic murmur

(E)   It indicates heart failure

140. Regarding ECG waveforms, all the following are true EXCEPT

(A)   the P wave reflects atrial depolarization

(B)   the QRS complex reflects ventricular depolarization

(C)   the U wave reflects atrial repolarization

(D)   the T wave reflects ventricular repolarization

(E)   the PR interval represents AV conduction time

141. While palpating a pulse you note that the pulse wave has two peaks. You auscultate the heart and are certain that there is only one heart beat for each two pulse waves. This finding is

(A)   pulsus alternans

(B)   dicrotic pulse

(C)   pulsus parvus et tardus

(D)   pulsus bigeminus

(E)   pulsus biferiens

142. Precipitating factors of acute atrial fibrillation include all the following EXCEPT

(A)   fever

(B)   pericarditis

(C)   hypertension

(D)   thyrotoxicosis

(E)   cardiac tamponade

143. All the following statements concerning the *c* wave of the venous pressure curve are true EXCEPT

(A) it occurs when the ventricle contracts
(B) it is decreased in tricuspid regurgitation
(C) it is caused by the bulging of the AV valves back into the atria
(D) it occurs simultaneously with the carotid pulse
(E) it is produced in part by the impact of the carotid artery against the jugular vein

144. All the following are signs or symptoms of hemorrhagic shock EXCEPT

(A) cool, clammy skin
(B) delayed capillary refill
(C) hypertension
(D) tachycardia
(E) pallor

145. All the following may be effects of arterial hypertension EXCEPT

(A) left ventricular hypertrophy
(B) pulmonary fibrosis
(C) angina pectoris
(D) cerebral hemorrhage
(E) renal failure

146. On physical examination of a patient with hypertension, which of the following is LEAST relevant?

(A) Paleness of skin
(B) Blood pressure of upper and lower extremities
(C) Supine and standing blood pressures
(D) Examination of optic fundi
(E) General appearance

147. The most common risk factor for dissection of the aorta is

(A) atherosclerosis
(B) diabetes mellitus
(C) aortic stenosis
(D) hypertension
(E) cigarette smoking

148. The most sensitive part of an examiner's hand to vibration is the

(A) fingertips
(B) pads of the finger
(C) wrist
(D) lateral edge
(E) medial edge

149. Regarding venous pulsations, all the following statements are true EXCEPT

(A) the venous pulse wave is a normal phenomenon

(B) venous pulsations are approximately one-sixteenth as strong as arterial pulsations

(C) the *a* wave results from atrial systole

(D) the *c* wave is caused by bulging of the mitral valve into the right atria

(E) the *v* wave is a result of atrial filling while the AV valves are closed

150. Which of the following statements regarding blood pressure is true?

(A) Precise limits for normal blood pressure are well established

(B) Hypertension is generally defined as a systolic blood pressure >140 mmHg or a diastolic blood pressure >90 mmHg

(C) A systolic blood pressure of <100 mmHg should be taken as normal

(D) A diastolic blood pressure of <60 mmHg should be taken as normal

(E) Blood pressure shows no change with age

151. True statements concerning findings of palpation of the chest wall include all the following EXCEPT

(A) a thrill may accompany an "innocent" murmur

(B) a left parasternal lift may be present in patients with right ventricular hypertrophy or a medially displaced point of maximal impulse (PMI) as in emphysema

(C) a laterally deviated, large PMI indicates left ventricular hypertrophy

(D) a systolic pulsation in the left second or third parasternal interspace indicates pulmonary hypertension

(E) a pulsation more sustained and medial than the PMI may indicate a dyskinetic ventricular wall segment

152. True statements regarding percussion of the chest include all the following EXCEPT

(A) percussion can be used to determine cardiac situs

(B) percussion can be used to ascertain cardiac size

(C) percussion has a margin of error of 1 cm

(D) the accuracy of percussion is unaffected by obesity

(E) many ways to percuss the heart are successful if used consistently

153. Choose the true statement concerning the second heart sound (S_2).

(A) It is best heard at the apex

(B) It is louder than S_1 at the apex

(C) It is normally made up of P_2 followed by A_2

(D) Inspiration increases the split of S_2

(E) Splitting is caused by increased filling of the left ventricle

154. All the following statements are true concerning paradoxical splitting of S_2 EXCEPT

(A) the split is longer during expiration

(B) the split may be due to shortening of left ventricular ejection time

(C) the split may be due to shortening of right ventricular ejection time

(D) aortic stenosis may cause a split S_2

(E) the split may be found rarely in uncomplicated hypertension

155. Wide, fixed splitting of S_2

(A) changes with respiration

(B) may be caused by either electrical or mechanical means

(C) is commonly caused by left bundle branch block or ventricular septal defect

(D) may be confused with a normal S_2 followed closely by an S_4

(E) may be caused by pulmonic valve insufficiency

156. True statements concerning gallops include all the following EXCEPT

(A) they are high-pitched sounds

(B) S_3 follows S_2 and is known as ventricular diastolic gallop

(C) S_4 precedes S_1 and is known as atrial diastolic gallop

(D) they are best heard using the bell of the stethoscope

(E) S_3 and S_4 may occur at the same time with rapid heart rates

157. All the following statements about S_3 and S_4 are true EXCEPT

(A) an S_3 gallop is caused by abnormal ventricular compliance

(B) an S_3 gallop may be found in some normal children

(C) an S_4 gallop is caused by blood from the atrial kick as it enters a ventricle with decreased compliance

(D) S_4 may be audible in normal persons

(E) an S_3 gallop has little diagnostic significance in congestive heart failure

158. Causes of continuous murmurs include all the following EXCEPT

(A) coronary arteriovenous fistula

(B) aortic stenosis

(C) patent ductus arteriosus

(D) cervical venous hum

(E) hepatic venous hum

159. Standing increases the murmur of

(A) tricuspid insufficiency
(B) aortic insufficiency
(C) mitral stenosis
(D) hypertrophic subaortic stenosis
(E) pulmonary stenosis

160. Squatting has which of the following cardiovascular effects?

(A) It decreases ventricular filling
(B) It increases the murmur of aortic insufficiency
(C) It decreases the murmur of a ventricular septal defect
(D) It decreases the murmur of mitral regurgitation
(E) It decreases a pulmonary flow murmur

161. Choose the correct statement regarding aortic insufficiency.

(A) It is a high-pitched, blowing, diastolic murmur
(B) It is best heard with the bell of the stethoscope
(C) The first heart sound is usually abnormal in patients with aortic insufficiency
(D) A decreased pulse pressure is usually found in patients with aortic insufficiency
(E) It is best heard at the apex of the heart

162. Aortic stenosis is correctly characterized by the statement that

(A) it is heard exclusively at the apex
(B) it is a systolic murmur
(C) it is a pansystolic murmur
(D) it has a flat configuration on phonocardiogram
(E) it rarely causes hypertrophy of the heart

163. True statements regarding mitral regurgitation include which of the following?

(A) It is a diastolic murmur
(B) It radiates only to the base of the heart
(C) It is best heard at the apex
(D) It begins after slight delay following S_2
(E) It lasts completely from S_2 to S_1

164. Which of the following statements is true of detection of abdominal aortic aneurysms (AAAs) by physical examination?

(A) AAAs are not detectable by physical examination
(B) Obesity reduces the ability to detect AAA on physical examination
(C) Most AAAs are detectable by physical examination
(D) Ninety-five percent of AAAs are palpable
(E) AAAs are overdiagnosed by physical examination

165. True statements about mitral stenosis include that

(A) it is a systolic murmur
(B) it is a holosystolic murmur
(C) it radiates widely throughout the precordium
(D) it is best heard at the apex with the bell of the stethoscope
(E) it has a pure timbre

166. All the following statements concerning tricuspid regurgitation are true EXCEPT

(A) it is a systolic murmur
(B) it is best heard at the left sternal border in the fourth and fifth interspaces
(C) it causes prominent c waves of the venous pulse in the neck
(D) inspiration decreases the murmur
(E) it does not radiate to the axilla

167. All the following are modifiable risk factors for myocardial infarction EXCEPT

(A) cigarette smoking
(B) hypertension
(C) age
(D) obesity
(E) elevated cholesterol level

Items 168–169

On examining a 51-year-old man who was just involved in a motor vehicle accident, you find that at the end of expiration his blood pressure is 130/90 mmHg and at the end of inspiration it is 110/92 mmHg.

168. Which of the following conditions is most likely?

(A) Cardiac tamponade
(B) Tetralogy of Fallot
(C) Atrial septal defect
(D) Left ventricular failure
(E) Aortic insufficiency

169. What is the name of the blood pressure changes observed in this man?

(A) Garrin-Frey phenomenon
(B) Pulsus alternans
(C) Pulsus paradoxus
(D) Hypovolemic shock
(E) A positive tilt test

170. On physical examination of a 21-year-old woman, you auscultate at the apex of her heart a low-pitched mid-to-late diastolic murmur with accentuation of S_1. Upon careful listening you notice a clicking sound just after S_2 and immediately preceding the rumbling murmur. The most likely condition is

(A) aortic insufficiency
(B) atrial myxoma
(C) mitral valve prolapse
(D) mitral valve stenosis
(E) patent foramen ovale

171. A 6-year-old boy presents to your clinic for a routine physical examination. His right arm blood pressure is 150/110 mmHg, while his left leg blood pressure is 80/60 mmHg. On auscultation a systolic murmur best heard over the mid-upper back is detected. You also find that his femoral pulses are delayed when compared with his brachial. An ECG shows left-axis deviation. The most likely diagnosis is

(A) patent ductus arteriosus
(B) ventricular septal defect
(C) coarctation of the aorta
(D) aortic stenosis
(E) mitral valve prolapse

172. A mother brings her 10-year-old son to your office because he lost consciousness the day before while running. She says that he has had similar episodes in the past and that he does not seem to be able to play as long as most of his friends. He has been observed squatting down periodically while in the midst of activity. On physical examination you detect a low-pitched systolic ejection murmur and find that the point of maximal impulse is deviated laterally. The most likely diagnosis is

(A) mitral valve stenosis
(B) aortic stenosis
(C) coarctation of the aorta
(D) aortic insufficiency
(E) patent ductus arteriosus

173. On physical examination of a 15-year-old boy, you find a blood pressure of 140/55 mmHg at rest. You also notice a large, well-healed scar over the medial aspect of his left thigh. On questioning he states that he acquired the scar by impaling his thigh on a large nail after falling. Auscultation of the scar reveals a bruit and there is a palpable thrill. Most likely the patient has

(A) premature atherosclerosis
(B) an arteriovenous fistula
(C) scar tissue compressing the femoral artery
(D) congenital duplication of the femoral artery
(E) a bone tumor

174. On physical examination of a 3-month-old child you detect a thrill and a machinery-type murmur at the left upper sternal border. A widened systemic pulse pressure and bounding peripheral pulses are also noted. Based on these findings the most probable diagnosis is

(A) familial hypercholesterolemia
(B) patent ductus arteriosus
(C) tetralogy of Fallot
(D) Marfan's syndrome
(E) aortic stenosis

175. You are called to evaluate a 56-year-old man with chest, jaw, and left arm pain. On physical examination you find an anxious, pale man who is uncomfortable on the examination table. He is perspiring heavily although his extremities are cool. At this point the most likely diagnosis would be

(A) gastric ulcer
(B) angina pectoris
(C) pneumonia
(D) acute myocardial infarct
(E) appendicitis

DIRECTIONS: Each group of questions below consists of lettered options followed by numbered items. For each numbered item, select the appropriate lettered option(s). Each lettered option may be used once, more than once, or not at all. **Choose exactly the number of options indicated following each item.**

Items 176–178

Match each of the venous pulse abnormalities with its causative disorder.

(A) Tricuspid regurgitation
(B) Atrial fibrillation
(C) Tricuspid stenosis
(D) Pulmonary hypertension
(E) Complete heart block

176. Large systolic *v* wave **(SELECT 1 DISORDER)**

177. Cannon *a* wave **(SELECT 1 DISORDER)**

178. Absent *a* wave **(SELECT 1 DISORDER)**

Items 179–183

Match the physical finding or symptom with the most likely disorder or condition.

(A) Malignant hypertension
(B) Abdominal aortic aneurysm
(C) Renal artery stenosis
(D) Hypercholesterolemia
(E) Deep venous thrombosis

179. Xanthoma **(SELECT 1 CONDITION)**

180. Papilledema **(SELECT 1 CONDITION)**

181. Abdominal bruit **(SELECT 1 CONDITION)**

182. Pulsatile mass in the abdomen **(SELECT 1 CONDITION)**

183. Pain in calf with flexion of the foot **(SELECT 1 CONDITION)**

Cardiovascular System

Answers

116. The answer is E. *(Isselbacher, 13/e, p 950.)* S_1 is made up of mitral valve closure followed by tricuspid valve closure. Ordinarily these occur so close together that S_1 is heard as a single sound. If right ventricular contraction is delayed (as in right bundle branch block), closure of the tricuspid valve occurs even longer after the mitral valve has closed, and S_1 is split.

117. The answer is C. *(Tintinalli, 4/e, p 188.)* In addition to chest discomfort, patients with acute myocardial infarction may complain of dyspnea, nausea, vomiting, and diaphoresis. Fatigue, lethargy, and confusion may be present but are more common in elderly patients.

118. The answer is E. *(Isselbacher, 13/e, p 950.)* The intensity of S_1 is influenced by the position of the mitral leaflets at the end of ventricular systole, the rate of the ventricular pressure pulse, the presence of disease of the mitral valve, and the amount of tissue, air, or fluid between the heart and the stethoscope. The wider the mitral valve leaflets are spread when the ventricle contracts, the louder S_1 will be. Increased atrioventricular flow, a shortened PR interval, or a shortened diastole all cause a wider spread between valves and thus a louder S_1. A loud S_1 in mitral stenosis usually signifies a pliable valve that remains open at the onset of isovolumetric contraction because of elevated left atrial pressure. In atrial fibrillation, the intensity of S_1 is variable because of the variable spread of the mitral valve leaflets when the ventricle contracts.

119. The answer is D. *(Isselbacher, 13/e, p 950.)* S_2 is caused by the closure of the aortic valve (A_2) followed by the closure of the pulmonary valve (P_2). For this reason, anything that would prolong right ventricular ejection would increase the split between A_2 and P_2. Inspiration increases venous return (decreased thoracic pressure) and thereby prolongs right ventricular ejection. Standing decreases venous return because of pooling of blood in the lower extremities caused by gravity.

120. The answer is E. *(Isselbacher, 13/e, pp 950–954.)* S_3 is a low-pitched sound that occurs early in diastole at the termination of the rapid-filling phase. It may be found in normal children or persons with large cardiac outputs. If found in older patients, it usually indicates ventricular decompensation. An S_3 is best heard with the bell of the stethoscope.

121. The answer is A. *(Isselbacher, 13/e, pp 950–954.)* S_4 is a low-pitched sound that occurs just prior to systole (just before S_1) and is associated with ventricular filling as a result of an effective atrial contraction. For this reason it is absent in patients with atrial fibrillation. The incidence of S_4 increases with age, but the significance of this finding in the absence of other heart disease remains controversial.

122. The answer is A. *(Isselbacher, 13/e, pp 950–954.)* A good rule of thumb is that the increased venous return of inspiration increases the murmurs of the right side of the heart and expiration increases the murmurs of the left side of the heart. The murmur of tricuspid regurgitation (holosystolic murmur at the lower left sternal border) is therefore increased by inspiration. Other clues to the diagnosis of tricuspid regurgitation are distended neck veins, prominent v waves, hepatomegaly, edema, and a positive hepatojugular reflux (pressure applied over the liver causes increased distention of the neck veins).

123. The answer is D. *(Isselbacher, 13/e, pp 1011–1036.)* The key word in this question is *rate*. A sinus arrhythmia is the only answer that directly affects rate. In pulsus paradoxus the blood pressure decreases (more than 10 mmHg) with inspiration and is associated with compromised cardiac filling. Pulsus paradoxus is usually associated with pericardial disease, especially cardiac tamponade. Pulsus alternans also is a drop in the blood pressure, but it is associated with every other beat. The mechanism is unknown but it is usually due to an altered left ventricular contractile force.

124. The answer is D. *(Isselbacher, 13/e, pp 950–954.)* Murmurs are caused by turbulent flow of blood. They are graded I to VI. A grade I murmur is so faint that it escapes detection except by the most highly trained persons and then only after they listen to several cardiac cycles. A grade III murmur is not loud, but should not be missed by even an inexperienced examiner. A grade VI murmur is so prominent that it can be heard without the stethoscope's contacting the chest wall.

125. The answer is B. *(Isselbacher, 13/e, pp 950–954.)* Since sounds are auscultated throughout the cardiac cycle, the best diagnosis is pericarditis. The scratchy nature of the sounds represents the heart's movement against the inflamed pericardium. In mitral valve prolapse the most common finding is a mid-to-late systolic click followed by a high-pitched late systolic crescendo-decrescendo murmur. Coarctation of the aorta typically causes a midsystolic murmur that, if severe, may become continuous throughout the cardiac cycle. It would then be important to look for some of the other signs of coarctation, such as delayed femoral pulse and enlarged collateral vessels, to differentiate between these two types of continuous murmurs. Pneumonias generally do not affect the heart sounds. Rales, rhonchi, and decreased breath sounds in the lung fields may indicate the presence of a pneumonia.

126. The answer is A. *(Isselbacher, 13/e, pp 939–941.)* HDL is considered a protective factor against the development of atherosclerosis. Elevated cholesterol levels (>200 mg/dL) are associated with an increased risk of development of atherosclerosis and ischemic heart disease. Diabetics have at least a twofold increase in the incidence of myocardial infarction. This suggests a role for hyperglycemia in atherogenesis. Smoking is one of the most potent risk factors for atherosclerosis. Statistical evidence demonstrates a mean increase of 70 percent in the death rate in men who smoke one pack of cigarettes per day. Hypertension is also an important risk factor, and the risk increases proportionally with the high blood pressure. Ischemic heart disease is five times more common in men with blood pressures >160/95 mmHg when compared with normotensive men (pressures <140/90 mmHg).

127. The answer is D. *(Isselbacher, 13/e, pp 1011–1036.)* Atrial fibrillation (AF) is a common dysrhythmia that can occur in normal people, especially during emotional stress, after surgery or exercise, or following an alcoholic binge. It is also seen in hypoxia, hypercapnia, and in some metabolic and hemodynamic disturbances. Chronic AF occurs in patients with cardiovascular disease, especially rheumatic heart disease, mitral valve disease, hypertensive cardiomyopathy, atrial septal defect, and chronic lung disease. AF may be the first finding in thyrotoxicosis. Whenever the pulse is felt to be irregularly irregular, AF is almost always the diagnosis.

128. The answer is C. *(Isselbacher, 13/e, p 1142.)* Varicose veins are a common complaint, especially in women. They are most commonly found in the superficial veins of the lower extremities. Varicose veins are caused by valve incompetence in veins that connect the superficial venous system to the deep venous system. This leads to increased pressure in the superficial veins and subsequent dilatation. They have not been associated with heart disease. Varicosities rarely cause life-threatening problems, but they are not innocuous. Stasis dermatitis and skin ulceration are common complications of varicosities. Varicose veins often become calcified.

129. The answer is A. *(Tintinalli, 4/e, p 191.)* Many signs and symptoms may accompany pulmonary embolism. Pleuritic chest pain, tachypnea, and tachycardia are the most common signs and symptoms in pulmonary embolism.

130. The answer is D. *(Isselbacher, 13/e, pp 1066–1077.)* After acute myocardial infarction, CPK levels rise within the first 6 to 8 h, peak within 24 to 36 h, and return to normal in 36 to 48 h. AST levels rise within 8 h, peak at 36 h, and return to normal within 72 h. LDH levels peak in 3 to 4 days and return to normal over 14 days.

131. The answer is C. *(Isselbacher, 13/e, p 1079.)* Variant (Prinzmetal's) angina differs from stable (exertional) angina in that it usually occurs at rest. The onset is sudden and frightening and causes chest discomfort and shortness of breath. The pathophysiology is vasospasm of proximal epicardial coronary arteries, and most of the time there is atherosclerosis, which is the focus for the spasm.

132. The answer is C. *(Isselbacher, 13/e, pp 1046–1052.)* Rheumatic fever is an inflammatory disease that occurs as a delayed sequela to an infection with group A streptococci, usually pharyngitis. The Jones criteria are used when making the diagnosis of rheumatic fever. The presence of two major criteria or one major criterion and two minor criteria indicates a high probability that rheumatic fever is present, given the history of recent streptococcal infection. The major Jones criteria for rheumatic fever are endocarditis, chorea, erythema marginatum, subcutaneous nodules, and polyarthritis. The minor criteria are fever, malaise, abdominal pain, arthralgias, elevated sedimentation rate, leukocytosis, and a preceding streptococcal infection.

133. The answer is E. *(Isselbacher, 13/e, pp 948–949.)* The normal jugular venous pressure (JVP) reflects phasic pressure changes in the right atrium. It usually consists of two and sometimes three positive and two negative troughs. The *a* wave is caused by atrial contraction, which is represented by the P wave on ECG. Therefore, the *a* wave occurs just after the P wave and prior to the QRS complex. The other positive waves are the *c* and *v* waves. The negative waves are the *x* and *y* descents.

134. The answer is B. *(Isselbacher, 13/e, pp 948–949.)* The *a* wave is due to venous distention caused by atrial contraction. It is the most dominant wave, especially during inspiration. The *a* wave is not present in atrial fibrillation. Exaggerated *a* waves, known as "cannon" *a* waves, occur when the right atrium is contracting against increased resistance. They are most commonly seen with pulmonary hypertension or pulmonic stenosis, but they can also be seen with tricuspid stenosis.

135. The answer is B. *(Isselbacher, 13/e, 1116–1117.)* To make the diagnosis of hypertension, several elevated readings must be obtained. Of all the cases of hypertension, only 5 to 10 percent have a known etiology. Patients with hypertension die prematurely from several illnesses but especially heart diseases. Recognition and treatment may be the reason for reduction in cardiovascular mortality over the last 20 to 30 years.

136. The answer is B. *(Isselbacher, 13/e, pp 1214–1215.)* Emboli usually arise from the deep veins of the lower extremities and pelvis and are much more common after prolonged bed rest, immobilization, and a major operation. Many patients dying from pulmonary emboli have serious underlying medical conditions, such as cancer and congestive heart failure. Even though less than 10 percent of all emboli are fatal, 50,000 deaths each year in the U.S. are attributed to pulmonary embolism. The incidence of venous thrombosis increases during pregnancy and with the taking of birth control pills.

137. The answer is C. *(Isselbacher, 13/e, pp 1043–1044.)* In coarctation of the aorta the femoral pulse is weak because of the obstruction to flow in the aorta. This constriction is usually distal to the left subclavian artery. The pulse pressure typically is increased and the blood pressure in the legs is less than that in the arms. A chest x-ray may show notching of the ribs secondary to dilated collateral arteries.

138. The answer is C. *(Isselbacher, 13/e, pp 950–954.)* During a sustained Valsalva maneuver the thoracic pressure is greatly increased; therefore, the venous return drops, followed by a drop in the cardiac output. To compensate, the heart rate increases. In hypertrophic aortic stenosis, the decreased venous return decreases left ventricular volume; therefore, the outflow tract is smaller and the murmur louder.

139. The answer is D. *(Isselbacher, 13/e, pp 945–954.)* A precordial thrill is a palpable organic murmur that is best timed by palpation. It most likely accompanies some type of heart disease. Thrills should always be considered pathologic. The presence of a thrill characterizes a murmur as at least grade IV.

140. The answer is C. *(Isselbacher, 13/e, pp 954–966.)* In a normal ECG, the P wave represents atrial depolarization. The QRS complex reflects ventricular depolarization, while the T wave represents ventricular repolarization.

Atrial repolarization cannot be seen on a normal ECG because it is masked by the QRS complex (ventricular depolarization). The PR interval can be used as a measure of AV conduction time. A U wave is not normally present, and when it is, it most likely represents hypokalemia or ischemic heart disease.

141. The answer is E. *(Isselbacher, 13/e, p 948.)* Pulsus biferiens (biferious pulse) is seen in aortic regurgitation and in hypertrophic cardiomyopathy. In the latter, the first wave (percussion wave) is due to the rapid flow rate of initial contraction, and the second wave (tidal wave) is due to the slower rate of continued contraction. The dicrotic pulse has two palpable pulses, but one is in systole and the other in diastole. Pulsus bigeminus (bigeminal pulse) is an alteration in pulse amplitude that follows a ventricular premature beat. Pulsus alternans is a regular alternating pulse amplitude due to alternating left ventricular contractile force; it is usually seen with severe left ventricular decompensation. Pulsus parvus et tardus represents a delayed systolic peak. It is due to mechanical obstruction to left ventricular ejection and usually is associated with a coarse systolic thrill.

142. The answer is E. *(Isselbacher, 13/e, pp 1022–1023.)* There are many conditions that may predispose a patient to atrial fibrillation. Some of these are fever, pericarditis, hypertension, and thyrotoxicosis. Atrial fibrillation may also be seen in normal subjects in periods of stress, after surgery, and during exercise or alcohol intoxication.

143. The answer is B. *(Sapira, p 363.)* The *c* wave of the venous pressure curve occurs as a result of ventricular contraction, which forces the tricuspid valve back toward the atria as well as distorts the atrial cavity. For that reason it is simultaneous with the carotid pulse. If the tricuspid valve is incompetent, the *c* wave will be increased.

144. The answer is C. *(Tintinalli, 4/e, p 197.)* In the early phase of hemorrhagic shock, blood is shunted away from the skin and distal extremities, causing cool, clammy skin and delayed capillary refill. As the condition worsens, hypotension, tachycardia, decreased peripheral pulses, pallor, tachypnea, agitation, and decreased urine output are characteristic.

145. The answer is B. *(Isselbacher, 13/e, pp 1116–1118.)* Hypertension causes excess strain on the heart, which leads to left ventricular hypertrophy, and, as oxygen consumption increases, to angina pectoris. Cerebral hemorrhage also may occur as a result of elevated arterial blood pressure and the formation of microaneurysms (Charcot-Bouchard). There are many other complaints linked to hypertension: fatigue, dizziness, palpitations, proteinuria, hematuria, and others.

146. The answer is A. *(Isselbacher, 13/e, pp 1116–1117.)* On examination of a patient with hypertension, it is important to measure the blood pressure in all extremities with the patient supine and standing. In so doing, differences may be detected that lead to the diagnosis of secondary hypertension from coarctation or pheochromocytoma. Examination of the optic fundi may show hypertensive changes (hemorrhages, exudates, arteriovenous crossing changes) that would indicate the high blood pressure was long-standing. Paleness of skin has little to do with hypertension.

147. The answer is D. *(Isselbacher, 13/e, pp 1132–1133.)* Dissection of the aorta occurs when the intima is interrupted so that blood enters the wall of the aorta and separates its layers. It is almost always fatal if undiagnosed, but with prompt treatment the majority of patients survive. The most common risk factor is hypertension, but anything that weakens the media can lead to dissection of the aorta. Aortic dissection is a major cause of morbidity and mortality in Marfan's syndrome. The incidence of aortic dissection is increased when there is a congenital aortic valve anomaly or coarctation of the aorta and during the third trimester of pregnancy.

148. The answer is B. *(Seidel, 3/e, p 60.)* The palmar pads of the fingers are most sensitive to vibration. This can be demonstrated by placing a tuning fork alternately on the fingertips, lateral and medial margins, and palmar fingertip areas. For this reason, the palm of the hand should be used for cardiac palpation.

149. The answer is D. *(Seidel, 3/e, pp 415–418.)* The venous pressure curve is a normal phenomenon that can be demonstrated near the heart in any superficial vein, most commonly the external jugular veins. The *a* wave is produced by atrial contraction, and it would therefore be absent in atrial fibrillation. It is followed by the *c* wave, which is caused by the tricuspid valve's bulging backward at the beginning of systole. The *v* wave is produced by atrial filling.

150. The answer is B. *(Seidel, 3/e, pp 414–415.)* The limits for a normal blood pressure are not well established but are taken as a systolic pressure between 100 and 140 mmHg and a diastolic pressure of between 60 and 90 mmHg. Hypertension is generally accepted to be a systolic pressure >160 mmHg or a diastolic pressure >90 mmHg. Blood pressure generally increases with age.

151. The answer is A. *(Sapira, pp 284–285.)* Palpation of the chest can yield much useful information. A laterally displaced, enlarged PMI indicates left ventricular hypertrophy. A left parasternal lift may be due to right ventricular hypertrophy or a medially displaced PMI as in patients with emphysema. If a thrill is palpable, it indicates a pathologic murmur of grade IV or greater. Pulmonary hypertension may be detected by a left parasternal pulsation in the second or third intercostal spaces. Ventricular dyskinesia may be detected by palpation of a more medial and sustained pulsation than the PMI.

152. The answer is D. *(Sapira, p 286.)* Percussion of the heart is useful in determining cardiac situs and size. This has a practical application when a patient's heart appears enlarged on a chest x-ray. Remember that the heart is artificially enlarged on an anteroposterior projection. Percussion's margin of error is taken to be 1.0 cm. Obesity increases this error. Consistency is the key to success when percussing.

153. The answer is D. *(Sapira, p 293.)* S_2 consists of closure of the aortic valve (A_2) followed by that of the pulmonic valve (P_2). It is best heard at the base of the heart, where it is louder than S_1. Inspiration increases the split of S_2 by two mechanisms. First, there is delayed pulmonic valve closure, which is due to prolonged right ventricular ejection time from increased stroke volume. Second, inspiration increases the compliance of the pulmonary vasculature and thereby decreases the return of blood to the left heart and shortens its ejection time by the same mechanism.

154. The answer is B. *(Sapira, p 295.)* Paradoxical splitting of S_2 is caused by anything that delays A_2 or speeds up P_2 to the point where P_2 occurs prior to A_2. For this reason, expiration separates a paradoxical split longer by prolonging left ventricular ejection and shortening right ventricular ejection. Other causes are left bundle branch block, aortic stenosis, and rarely systemic hypertension. Each of these prolongs left ventricular outflow.

155. The answer is B. *(Sapira, pp 295–296.)* A wide, fixed split of S_2 occurs both in inspiration and expiration. It may be caused by a delayed closure of the pulmonic valve due to electrical means, such as a right bundle branch block, or mechanical means, such as pulmonic stenosis or overload as in atrial septal defect. It also may be caused by early aortic valve closure as in mitral insufficiency or ventricular septal defect with a left-to-right shunt (the latter also overloads the right ventricle). S_2 should not be confused with S_4, which is a lower-pitched sound and occurs in late diastole.

156. The answer is A. *(Sapira, pp 296–297.)* Gallops (S_3, S_4) are low-pitched sounds heard best with the bell of the stethoscope at the apex of the heart (if originating from the left ventricle) or at the left sternal border (if from the right ventricle). The heart sounds occur as S_1, S_2, S_3, S_4, but when heard they seem to be S_4, S_1, S_2, S_3. If the heart rate is rapid, S_3 and S_4 may occur simultaneously as diastole shortens. This is termed a summation gallop.

157. The answer is E. *(Sapira, pp 298–299.)* The ventricular gallop (S_3) usually indicates that ventricular compliance is abnormal. This is an extremely important sign in the diagnosis of congestive heart failure. It may sometimes be heard in completely normal young people. An atrial gallop (S_4) is due to the atrial kick of blood as it rushes into the ventricle that has poor compliance secondary to the stretch already placed on it by early diastolic filling. Audible fourth heart sounds have been detected in apparently healthy older persons.

158. The answer is B. *(Sapira, p 304.)* Continuous murmurs occupy both systole and diastole. They have the same pitch and timbre throughout. The most common continuous murmur, a cervical venous hum, emanates from the jugular veins. Its only significance is that it may be confused with a pathologic murmur. Aortic stenosis causes a systolic murmur.

159. The answer is D. *(Sapira, p 308.)* Standing decreases ventricular filling. Therefore, it increases the murmur of idiopathic hypertrophic subaortic stenosis (IHSS). It also increases the murmur of mitral valve prolapse in 74 percent of cases. Standing decreases all other murmurs.

160. The answer is B. *(Sapira, p 308.)* Squatting increases ventricular filling. Therefore, it increases blood flow through the heart and increases the murmurs of aortic insufficiency, ventricular septal defect, mitral regurgitation, and pulmonary flow.

161. The answer is A. *(Isselbacher, 13/e, pp 950–954.)* Aortic insufficiency is a high-pitched, blowing, diastolic murmur. It is best heard with the diaphragm in the second right or the third left interspace. The pulse pressure is increased in patients with aortic insufficiency because of the aortic regurgitation, which increases the systolic pressure.

162. The answer is B. *(Isselbacher, 13/e, pp 950–954.)* The murmur of aortic stenosis is systolic and is best heard at the second right interspace, but it also may be present anywhere anteriorly down to the apex, although not into the axilla. The murmur is a crescendo-decrescendo murmur and thus has a diamond shape on the phonocardiogram. It begins slightly after S_1 and ends slightly prior to S_2. The outflow of the left ventricle is inhibited; therefore, left ventricular hypertrophy is often present.

163. The answer is C. *(Sapira, pp 300, 316.)* Mitral regurgitation causes a holosystolic murmur best heard at the apex of the heart. It radiates characteristically into the axilla. Chronic rheumatic heart disease is often the cause of mitral regurgitation, but other causes include a congenital anomaly, myocardial infarction, infective endocarditis, or any condition that results in left ventricular dilation to the extent that the mitral valve leaflets incompletely oppose each other when closed.

164. The answer is B. *(Chervu, Surgery 117:454, 1995.)* Early detection of abdominal aortic aneurysms (AAAs) has been advocated to decrease the high mortality of ruptured AAAs. In a study of 243 patients with AAAs, only 38 percent were detected by physical examination (PE). Forty-three percent of patients with AAAs detected on radiologic examination had palpable AAAs and should have been detected on PE. Twenty-three percent of AAAs were not palpable on PE, even when the diagnosis was known. Obese patients had only 15 percent of AAAs detected by PE, and only 33 percent were palpable.

165. The answer is D. *(Sapira, pp 300, 320.)* The murmur of mitral stenosis is diastolic. It is best heard at the apex and radiates minimally. Since it is a rumbling, low-pitched, crescendo-decrescendo murmur, it is best heard using the bell of the stethoscope.

166. The answer is D. *(Sapira, pp 300, 322.)* Tricuspid regurgitation causes a systolic murmur best heard at the left sternal border in the fourth and fifth interspaces. It does not radiate to the axilla. The regurgitated blood causes prominent systolic waves in the jugular veins. Inspiration increases the murmur of tricuspid regurgitation.

167. The answer is C. *(Emergency Cardiac Care Committee, JAMA 268: 2174, 1992.)* Modifiable risk factors for myocardial infarction include cigarette smoking, hypertension, elevated cholesterol level, lack of exercise, obesity, stress, and diabetes. Risk factors that cannot be modified include heredity, male gender, race, and age.

168–169. The answers are 168-A, 169-C. *(Isselbacher, 13/e, pp 1096–1097.)* Cardiac tamponade is the accumulation of fluid in the pericardial sac in amounts sufficient to cause obstruction of blood flow back to the heart. Tam-

ponade may follow trauma, surgery, and many other conditions. Pulsus paradoxus is a condition in which the systolic blood pressure falls by more than 10
mmHg during inspiration. It may also be seen in severe asthma or COPD.

170. The answer is D. *(Isselbacher, 13/e, pp 1052–1056.)* Mitral stenosis
is characterized by an opening snap just prior to a low-pitched, rumbling diastolic murmur. Mitral regurgitation is a systolic murmur. Aortic insufficiency
is a high-pitched diastolic murmur.

171. The answer is C. *(Isselbacher, 13/e, pp 1043–1044.)* Coarctation of
the aorta is a narrowing of the aorta usually just distal to the origin of the ductus arteriosus and subclavian artery. Headaches, epistaxis, cold extremities,
and claudication may occur. Absent, delayed, or markedly diminished femoral
pulses also may be found. The low arterial pressure in the lower limbs in the
face of hypertension in the arm is also a clue toward the diagnosis.

172. The answer is B. *(Isselbacher, 13/e, pp 1059–1061.)* Aortic stenosis
may exist for several years before becoming clinically significant. There are
three cardinal symptoms of aortic stenosis: dyspnea on exertion, syncope, and
angina pectoris. The murmur is a rough, low-pitched systolic murmur usually
heard at the base of the heart. The apex beat is usually displaced laterally as
a reflection of left ventricular hypertrophy.

173. The answer is B. *(Isselbacher, 13/2, pp 951–954.)* An acquired arteriovenous fistula may be diagnosed by the presence of a continuous murmur
and a palpable thrill over an area of previous trauma. The large pulse pressure
is an indication that a large portion of the cardiac output is bypassing the systemic vascular resistance through the fistula.

174. The answer is B. *(Isselbacher, 13/e, p 1042.)* Patent ductus arteriosus
is a condition in which the ductus arteriosus fails to close properly after birth.
Physical examination will reveal a characteristic machinery-type murmur at
the left upper sternal border. The runoff of blood through the ductus causes
the widened pulse pressure and the bounding peripheral pulses.

175. The answer is D. *(Isselbacher, 13/e, p 1066.)* Patients suffering from
an acute myocardial infarction are typically anxious and restless secondary to
extreme pain. This pain may radiate from the occipital area to the umbilicus,
but most commonly can be found in the central portion of the chest or epigastrium or both. Pallor, perspiration, and coolness of the extremities are
commonly observed.

176–178. The answers are 176-A, 177-E, 178-B. *(Isselbacher, 13/e, pp 952–953, 1064.)* When the tricuspid valve is incompetent, ventricular contraction forces blood retrograde through the valve and forms a large systolic *v* wave in the venous pressure curve. This also obliterates the *x* descent and results in the single large systolic wave.

Any time the right atrium contracts against a closed tricuspid valve (as may occur in complete heart block), cannon *a* waves will be present. These may occur regularly as in junctional rhythm or irregularly as in complete heart block.

The *a* wave of the venous pressure curve is caused by atrial contraction. In fibrillation there are no organized atrial contractions and therefore no *a* waves.

179–183. The answers are 179-D, 180-A, 181-C, 182-B, 183-E. *(Isselbacher, 13/e, pp 105, 106, 302, 1132-1133, 1216, 2064, 2068, A4-4.)* A xanthoma is a yellowish nodule deposited in the skin. It is usually accompanied by an elevated blood cholesterol level. Xanthomas are especially prominent in familial hypercholesterolemia.

Papilledema is a swelling of the optic nerve and can be detected on funduscopic examination. Its presence, accompanied by retinal hemorrhages and exudates, rather than the absolute blood pressure level defines malignant hypertension.

Auscultation for an abdominal bruit that originates from stenotic renal arteries is an important part of the physical examination of a patient with hypertension. If present, a bruit is best heard just to the right or left of the midline above the umbilicus or in the flanks.

A pulsatile mass in the abdomen suggests the diagnosis of abdominal aortic aneurysm. A cross-table lateral abdominal x-ray may also suggest the diagnosis with curvilinear calcifications in the wall of the aneurysm. The diagnosis should be confirmed by ultrasound, which can delineate the size of the aorta and thickness of its walls.

Pain at the back of the knee or calf with dorsiflexion of the foot is Homans' sign. Presence of this sign suggests venous thrombosis of the leg. The sign is very inaccurate and the diagnosis of deep vein thrombosis should be established by other means, such as venography or Doppler ultrasound.

Thorax

DIRECTIONS: Each item below contains a question or incomplete statement followed by suggested responses. Select the **one best** response to each question.

184. A 50-year-old man with a 60-pack-year history of smoking presents with what appears to be enlarged and spongy fingertips that are slightly blue in color. Of the following, which is the most likely disease?

(A) Graves' disease
(B) Ulcerative colitis
(C) Crohn's disease
(D) Biliary cirrhosis
(E) Bronchogenic carcinoma

185. When two vertebrae prominens are felt, the lower one is

(A) C6
(B) C7
(C) C8
(D) T1
(E) T2

186. Wheezing is LEAST likely to be associated with which of the following?

(A) Congestive heart failure
(B) Paroxysmal nocturnal dyspnea
(C) Asthma
(D) Pneumonia
(E) Pulmonary embolism

187. A 56-year-old woman with a history of a 15-pound weight loss in the last 5 weeks complains that her meals are getting stuck in her "chest," and not only has this symptom been getting progressively worse, the feeling persists throughout the day. The most probable diagnosis is

(A) lower esophageal ring
(B) reflux esophagitis
(C) esophageal carcinoma
(D) paraesophageal hiatal hernia
(E) autonomic nervous system dysfunction

188. A 35-year-old woman with a history of type I diabetes mellitus is brought to the emergency room after not taking her routine insulin. The most likely type of respiration that she would be experiencing is

(A) Biot's
(B) severe panting
(C) Kussmaul's
(D) Cheyne-Stokes
(E) periodic

189. A 60-year-old man presents to your clinic with an 80-pack-year history of cigarette smoking, has an increased anteroposterior thickness of the thorax, and suffers from exertional dyspnea. He most likely suffers from

(A) chylothorax
(B) bronchiectasis
(C) panlobular emphysema
(D) lung abscess
(E) bronchial adenoma

190. A patient with pneumonia would most likely exhibit which of the following?

(A) Decreased fremitus and hyperresonance to percussion
(B) Increased fremitus and dullness to percussion
(C) Increased fremitus and hyperresonance to percussion
(D) Decreased fremitus and dullness to percussion
(E) Normal fremitus and hyperresonance to percussion

191. A 55-year-old man with an 80-pack-year smoking history would most likely have what type of respiratory pattern?

(A) Biot's
(B) Sighing
(C) Cheyne-Stokes
(D) Rapid and shallow
(E) Kussmaul's

192. A 22-year-old woman with a history of hypertension, use of oral contraceptives, and sickle cell anemia was involved in a motorcycle accident and is recovering from massive reconstructive surgery to her right leg. During her second week in traction, she develops tachypnea and tachycardia. Auscultation reveals a pleural friction rub, and roentgenographic findings show a raised left diaphragm and basilar atelectasis. The most likely diagnosis is

(A) bacterial pneumonia
(B) pneumothorax
(C) pulmonary embolism
(D) neurogenic shock
(E) hemorrhagic shock

193. A regular visitor to your emergency room presents in his usual inebriated state and is coughing up a foul-smelling sputum. Before collapsing he states, "Mr. Blue got the flu." The most likely diagnosis is

(A) stricture due to ingestion of lye
(B) pneumothorax due to blunt trauma
(C) spontaneous pneumothorax
(D) lung abscess secondary to aspiration
(E) bronchogenic carcinoma

194. True statements about idiopathic pulmonary fibrosis include all the following EXCEPT

(A) its peak incidence is in the fifth and sixth decades
(B) it was previously known as the Hamman-Rich syndrome
(C) it is more common in females
(D) it presents initially with exertional dyspnea
(E) x-ray films usually show evidence of fibrosis

195. Patients with centrilobular emphysema often have all the following EXCEPT

(A) a long history of steadily worsening dyspnea
(B) evidence of increased lung volume on x-ray
(C) a history of smoking
(D) a genetic deficiency of α_1-antitrypsin
(E) increased anteroposterior diameter ("barrel chest")

196. Which of the following variables in the history and physical examination is LEAST consistent with the diagnosis of chronic obstructive pulmonary disease (COPD)?

(A) History of smoking
(B) History of prior diagnosis of COPD
(C) Increased breath sounds
(D) Decreased peak flow

197. Adult respiratory distress syndrome (ARDS) has all the following characteristics EXCEPT

(A) it causes cyanosis
(B) it most frequently occurs secondary to sepsis or trauma
(C) it will have "wet" rales upon auscultation
(D) it will cause tachypnea
(E) it usually resolves without treatment

198. Pulmonary embolism has all the following characteristics EXCEPT

(A) it is associated with prolonged bed rest
(B) most emboli arise from thrombi originating in the right cardiac chambers
(C) it is associated with congestive heart failure
(D) it is associated with fracture of the femur
(E) it may cause sudden death

199. Auscultation of normal breath sounds of the chest demonstrates

(A) vesicular breath sounds that are high-pitched
(B) bronchial breath sounds heard over the trachea
(C) bronchovesicular breath sounds heard over the apices
(D) bronchial breath sounds that are the lowest in pitch and intensity
(E) maximal intensity at the lung bases toward the end of the expiratory phase

200. Which of the following statements regarding vocal resonance is true?

(A) Bronchophony is defined as greater clarity and decreased loudness in the spoken word

(B) Egophony is characterized by decreased intensity of the spoken word and a nasal quality (*e*'s become stuffy, broad *a*'s).

(C) There is decreased intensity of vocal resonance in emphysema

(D) Whispered pectoriloquy can occur when there is tympany to percussion

(E) When large accumulations of fluid compress the lower portion of the lung, voice sounds have a nasal quality over the lower lung

201. Croup is correctly characterized by which of the following statements?

(A) The inflammation is epiglottic

(B) It is associated with a rough, stridorous cough

(C) Girls are more often infected

(D) It is seldom associated with labored breathing

(E) It occurs most frequently in the teen-age years

202. Select the most accurate statement about epiglottitis.

(A) It resolves spontaneously

(B) The epiglottis appears pale and boggy

(C) It occurs most frequently between the ages of 1 and 3

(D) It has a sudden onset with rapid progression

(E) Diagnosis is obtained by a simple examination with a tongue blade

203. Which of the following statements concerning inspection of the thorax is true?

(A) During the third trimester the costal angle increases to 180°

(B) In the third trimester respirations can increase by 20 per minute and each will be more shallow

(C) In kyphosis there is flattening of the thoracic curvature and increased curvature in the lumbar spine

(D) Cystic fibrosis can cause a barrel chest

(E) Inspection begins when the patient's chest has been fully exposed

204. Which of the following statements regarding anatomic landmarks in the healthy patient is true?

(A) Posteriorly, the apices of the lungs rise to C7

(B) On deep inspiration, the lower lung borders reach L1

(C) On forced expiration, the lower lung borders rise to T8

(D) The trachea divides into right and left main bronchi just below the manubriosternal joint (sternal angle)

(E) The trachea is just to the right of midline

205. Tension pneumothorax can be described by which of the following statements?

(A) It can occur spontaneously without trauma

(B) Breath sounds and percussion are faint

(C) Deviation of the trachea is toward the affected side

(D) Air enters the thorax on expiration and communicates with the lung

(E) It demands intubation for relief

206. Smoking is known to be a risk factor for the increased incidence of all the following EXCEPT

(A) peptic ulcer

(B) centrilobular emphysema

(C) ectopic pregnancy

(D) carcinoma of the bladder

(E) laryngeal carcinoma

207. A man was stabbed and arrived at the emergency room within 30 min. You notice that the trachea is deviated away from the side of the chest that suffered the puncture. Which of the following would you find upon physical examination of the traumatized side?

(A) Increased fremitus

(B) Increased breath sounds

(C) Dullness to percussion

(D) Hyperresonant percussion

(E) Wheezing and stridor

208. A patient has a 1-week history of upper respiratory tract infection and is now complaining of fever, chills, cough, and thick sputum. Physical findings suggestive of pneumonia may include all the following EXCEPT

(A) increased tactile fremitus

(B) rales or rhonchi

(C) egophony

(D) tympanic percussion

(E) bronchial breath sounds

209. There was an explosion of a high-pressure phosgene storage tank at a government facility. It is well known that phosgene is not an upper-airway irritant. The first victims arrived at the emergency room within 15 min of the explosion. At this time they will most likely manifest all the following EXCEPT

(A) wheezing

(B) shortness of breath

(C) epiglottitis

(D) diffuse, moist rales

(E) nausea and dizziness

210. A patient with a history of hypertension is diagnosed as having congestive heart failure (CHF). Physical examination may reveal all the following EXCEPT

(A) lateral and downward displacement of the apical impulse
(B) a summation gallop
(C) fine, moist apical rales
(D) cardiomegaly
(E) increased heart rate

211. A mother brings her 4-year-old boy to your clinic, and she appears to be quite concerned with the boy's chest deformity. Upon exposure of the chest, you note a marked depression of the sternum below the clavicular-manubrial junction. All the following are true about his condition EXCEPT

(A) as the child develops, kyphoscoliosis may occur
(B) there may be pulmonary dysfunction
(C) this condition is called *pectus excavatum*
(D) there may be reduction in cardiac output
(E) this is a midline deformity, and you must do further examination to look for other midline defects

212. Which of the following is a characteristic finding in pleural effusion?

(A) Increased pleuritic pain
(B) Increased tactile fremitus to the spoken voice
(C) Lessened friction rub
(D) Invariably increased breath sounds
(E) Increased egophony

213. A 7-year-old boy who had had a mild upper respiratory tract infection for 2 days without fever or change in level of activity awakens with a temperature of 39.7°C (103.5°F), lassitude, and anorexia. He soon struggles to breathe and his parents bring him to the emergency room. On physical examination his vital signs include a pulse of 150 beats per minute and respiratory rate of 36 breaths per minute. The child is holding his arms around the back of a chair and exerting a great effort to breathe. He has a mucoid rhinorrhea, and auscultation reveals high-pitched breath sounds in all lung fields during expiration. The most appropriate diagnosis is

(A) epiglottitis
(B) asthma
(C) laryngotracheobronchitis
(D) tonsillitis
(E) pneumonia

214. A 4-year-old boy is brought to the emergency room soon after developing a fever of 39.44°C (103°F) and complaining to his mother that "it hurts to swallow." His voice sounds "weak and throaty." The boy has increasing difficulty with breathing, and it appears to the mother that "he can't get air in." Vital signs include a pulse of 156 beats per minute and a respiratory rate of 36 breaths per minute. The child appears anxious, his face is flushed, and he has saliva coming out of his mouth. He is holding his neck in an immobile, rigid manner. On auscultation, there is a very loud, high-pitched sound with each inspiration, heard best over the neck. The most appropriate diagnosis is

(A)   asthma
(B)   epiglottitis
(C)   laryngotracheobronchitis
(D)   tonsillitis
(E)   pneumonia

215. A 3-year-old girl has had a low-grade fever, "raspy" cough, and clear rhinorrhea for 3 days. She does not improve and begins to develop difficulty breathing. Vital signs include a temperature of 39.72°C (103.5°F), a pulse of 160 beats per minute, and a respiratory rate of 36 breaths per minute. Auscultation reveals bilateral rhonchi, wheezing, and some mild stridor. The most appropriate diagnosis is

(A)   asthma
(B)   epiglottitis
(C)   laryngotracheobronchitis
(D)   tonsillitis
(E)   pneumonia

216. A 2-year-old boy is having trouble breathing. The mother states that he has had a cough since he was born, and that this visit for breathing difficulty is one of many. The neonatal history includes that the boy did not defecate for quite some time after delivery. You chart his growth and find that he is in less than the fifth percentile. With this information, what additional test are you going to order?

(A)   HIV test
(B)   Immunoglobulin electro-phoresis
(C)   Urine drug screen
(D)   Sweat test
(E)   Rectal biopsy

217. A 13-year-old boy who is in a very worried state of mind says that he is growing breasts and that they hurt. He states that he has been growing taller this past year, and that he has no other complaints. On physical examination you note some acne on his face, that his testes and phallus are appropriate for age, that his scrotum is reddened with thinning of the skin, and that he has fine, sparse pubic hair. Your working diagnosis is

(A) normal puberty
(B) Klinefelter's syndrome
(C) pituitary tumor
(D) adrenal tumor
(E) gonadal tumor

218. A 5-year-old girl is brought to the emergency room by her camp counselor. The patient had suddenly developed a cough and noisy breathing while playing a late-night game of hide-and-seek. She usually takes some kind of medicine, but has not since arriving at camp. She is in respiratory distress and actively using her accessory muscles. Her respiration is harsh with wheezing in both phases. The expiratory phase is prolonged, and there is tachypnea and tachycardia. You diagnose the patient as having

(A) foreign body obstruction
(B) epilepsy
(C) asthma
(D) carcinoid tumor
(E) chronic bronchitis

219. A 4-hour-old girl had been doing fine until the nurses attempted to challenge-feed the newborn. She became cyanotic during the attempt, but improved with a return to crying when the attempt at feeding was discontinued. The most likely diagnosis is

(A) hyaline membrane disease
(B) choanal atresia
(C) transient tachypnea of the newborn
(D) meconium aspiration syndrome
(E) tracheoesophageal fistula

220. All the following present with stridor EXCEPT

(A) laryngotracheal bronchitis
(B) infectious croup
(C) foreign body aspiration
(D) bronchial asthma
(E) epiglottitis

221. The most common cause of airway obstruction is

(A) a foreign body
(B) edema
(C) the tongue
(D) bleeding
(E) trauma

222. A 6-week-old girl is constantly coughing. She is afebrile and began coughing about 10 days ago with increasing regularity. There were no complications during the pregnancy, labor, or delivery. When the infant was 10 days old a mild conjunctivitis developed, which responded successfully to 10 days of topical erythromycin. The respiratory rate is 55 breaths per minute, there are supraclavicular and intercostal retractions, the cough is paroxysmal and staccato in character, and auscultation reveals bilateral rales. Chest roentgenograph shows a diffuse interstitial infiltrate. The most likely diagnosis is

(A) group B streptococcal sepsis
(B) chlamydial pneumonia
(C) pertussis
(D) respiratory syncytial viral pneumonia
(E) aspiration pneumonia

223. A patient presents complaining that he "can't breathe." Of the following, which is LEAST likely to help you assess acute respiratory distress?

(A) Pursed-lip breathing
(B) Cyanosis
(C) Diaphoresis
(D) Respiratory rate
(E) Accessory muscle use

224. A 14-year-old boy presents with a history of chronic sinusitis and frequent pneumonias. You note that the heart sounds are best heard on the right side of the chest, and percussion shows the heart to be right-sided. The most likely diagnosis is

(A) cystic fibrosis
(B) Kartagener's syndrome
(C) empyema
(D) pulmonary dysplasia
(E) tracheoesophageal fistula

225. A 58-year-old woman complains of the gradual worsening of severe, burning, chest pain that is unilateral and linear in character. Examination reveals a low-grade fever and a tender, reddened band around the right chest. The most likely diagnosis is

(A) pericarditis
(B) rheumatoid lung disease
(C) contact dermatitis
(D) rib fracture
(E) shingles

226. Which of the following might suggest the diagnosis of chronic obstructive pulmonary disease (COPD)?

(A) Barrel chest
(B) Stridor
(C) Dullness to percussion of the chest
(D) Biot's respiration
(E) Increased tactile fremitus

DIRECTIONS: Each group of questions below consists of lettered options followed by numbered items. For each numbered item, select the appropriate lettered option(s). Each lettered option may be used once, more than once, or not at all. **Choose exactly the number of options indicated following each item.**

Items 227–231

Match each mediastinal mass with the most likely radiographic finding.

(A) Gas
(B) Tooth
(C) Anterior calcification
(D) Phlebolith
(E) Grade 5 density

227. Teratoma **(SELECT 1 FINDING)**

228. Hemangioma **(SELECT 1 FINDING)**

229. Thymoma **(SELECT 1 FINDING)**

230. Hiatal hernia **(SELECT 1 FINDING)**

231. Foreign object **(SELECT 1 FINDING)**

Items 232–236

For each condition below, select the most likely respiratory pattern.

(A) Cheyne-Stokes respiration
(B) Kussmaul's respiration
(C) Biot's respiration
(D) Hyperventilation
(E) Rapid, shallow breathing with prolonged expiration

232. Severely increased intracranial pressure **(SELECT 1 PATTERN)**

233. Sleep in children and older adults **(SELECT 1 PATTERN)**

234. Severe diabetic acidosis **(SELECT 1 PATTERN)**

235. Massive liver enlargement **(SELECT 1 PATTERN)**

236. An 80-pack-year smoking history in a 50-year-old man **(SELECT 1 PATTERN)**

Items 237–241

Match each clinical presentation with the correct breast disease.

(A) Breast cancer, classic presentation
(B) Paget's disease
(C) Inflammatory breast carcinoma
(D) Intraductal papilloma
(E) Fibroadenoma

237. A mobile mass with well-defined margins in a woman under 30 years of age

238. Hard, circumscribed, fixed, edematous mass with a *peau d'orange* appearance of the overlying skin

239. Bloody discharge from the nipple, without a palpable mass

240. Increased local temperature, redness, and a visible erysipeloid margin

241. Eczematoid changes in the nipple, including itching, burning, oozing, and bleeding

DIRECTIONS: Each group of questions below consists of four lettered options followed by a set of numbered items. For each numbered item select

A	if the item is associated with	(A) only
B	if the item is associated with	(B) only
C	if the item is associated with	**both** (A) and (B)
D	if the item is associated with	**neither** (A) nor (B)

Each lettered option may be used **once, more than once, or not at all.**

Items 242–244

(A) Bacterial pneumonia
(B) Viral pneumonia
(C) Both
(D) Neither

242. Abrupt onset

243. Rusty sputum

244. Chills

Items 245–249

(A) Epiglottitis
(B) Viral croup
(C) Both
(D) Neither

245. Most common between 3 months and 3 years of age

246. Fall and winter occurrence most common

247. Acute onset

248. Fever usually greater than 39.44°C (103°F)

249. Typical presence of an extremely sore throat

Thorax

Answers

184. The answer is E. *(Sapira, p 258.)* Clubbing, a hypertrophic osteo-arthropathy, may be seen in a multitude of diseases, such as congenital cyanotic heart disease, bacterial endocarditis, biliary cirrhosis, Crohn's disease, severe ulcerative colitis, myelogenous leukemia, chronic renal failure, and Graves' disease. When clubbing is found in association with cyanosis, however, often the most important underlying condition to be aware of is bronchogenic carcinoma. Clubbing is detected as follows: Observe the angle between the nail bed and the base of the finger, the ungual-phalangeal angle (Lovibond's angle). This should be less than 180°. Some physicians have the patient place the right and left fingers against each other, knuckle to knuckle and fingernail tip to fingernail tip. If there is no abnormality of the angle, a definite rhombus will be seen between the distal phalanges; however, if Lovibond's angle is greater than 180°, no such rhombus will be seen.

185. The answer is D. *(Moore, 3/e, pp 33, 331, 427, 783.)* The vertebra prominens is the spinous process of C7, and it is most readily seen and palpated with the patient's head bent forward. If two prominences are felt, the lower one is the spinous process of T1. It is difficult to use this as a guide to counting the ribs posteriorly because the spinous processes from T4 down project obliquely and thus overlie the rib *below* the number of its vertebra. There are only seven cervical vertebrae.

186. The answer is D. *(Seidel, 3/e, pp 344–347.)* Classically, wheezing is associated with small airway obstruction, as can occur with bronchial asthma (especially postexercise wheezing), endobronchial tumors and granulomas (which usually present with unilateral wheezing), foreign body aspiration (depending on the size of the foreign body and the reaction of the airway, though foreign bodies usually do not lodge in the small airways), and acute bronchitis. In congestive heart failure, left ventricular failure can bring about symptoms that are known collectively as cardiac asthma, which includes paroxysmal nocturnal dyspnea. Another important cause of wheezing is pulmonary embolism, which presents with acute onset of dyspnea, pleuritic chest pain, and a cough. Pneumonia, without bronchoconstriction, is not usually associated with wheezing.

187. The answer is C. *(Isselbacher, 13/e, pp 206, 207, 1383.)* Esophageal dysphagia usually presents as a sticking sensation. When it is intermittent, it is usually associated with a lower esophageal ring; when it is progressive, it is usually due to a tumor. Regurgitation may occur minutes to hours after a meal. Patients find that they have to chew their food more thoroughly and that they require increased fluid consumption to "wash the food down." The length of time taken to consume a meal is prolonged.

188. The answer is C. *(Berkow, 16/e, pp 1022, 1106, 1122.)* Diabetic ketoacidosis (blood pH 7.2 or lower) induces a distinctive respiratory pattern known as Kussmaul's breathing, which consists of slow and deep respirations that increase the tidal volume. Since the breathing capacity is not hampered, the patient rarely complains of dyspnea. The uremic patient will often complain of dyspnea due to the severe panting brought on by combinations of acidosis, heart failure, pulmonary edema, and anemia. Cerebral lesions, such as intracranial hemorrhage, are often associated with intense hyperventilation that is sometimes noisy and stertorous and also has unpredictable, irregular periods of apnea alternating with periods in which four or five breaths of similar depth are taken; this breathing pattern is known as Biot's respiration. Periodic, or Cheyne-Stokes, respiration has a rhythmic, alternating, gradually changing pattern of apnea and hyperpnea that may be of CNS or cardiac origin. Slowing of the circulation, as happens in heart failure, is the cause most often seen. Both acidosis and hypoxia affect the respiratory centers in the medulla oblongata, and together they can create the respiratory pattern associated with Cheyne-Stokes.

189. The answer is C. *(Isselbacher, 13/e, pp 1197–1206.)* The increased anteroposterior thickness of the thorax indicates the presence of a "barrel-chest," which in association with a smoking history and exertional dyspnea is a classic presentation of emphysema. Emphysema due to cigarette smoking nearly always begins as centrilobular emphysema, but as the pack-years increase the emphysema progresses to panlobular in nature. With bronchiectasis there is usually a history of repeated episodes of pneumonia or bronchitis, and a classic presentation would be the long-term production of a foul-smelling sputum. Chylothorax commonly presents secondary to chest trauma or lymphoma or as a postsurgical complication, and the pleural effusion is milky, has normal cholesterol and increased triglyceride content, and stains with Sudan III. Lung abscess occurs frequently in alcoholics from aspiration following unconsciousness, and common complaints include halitosis, foul-smelling sputum, and fever. With a bronchial adenoma there is a paucity of physical findings, but the patient may present with wheezing, recurrent bouts of pneumonia, or hemoptysis.

190. The answer is B. *(Sapira, p 250.)* *Fremitus* refers to vibrations that are perceived in a tactile, nonacoustic manner; thus, it is often referred to redundantly as *tactile fremitus.* Pneumonia can be caused by bacteria, fungi, or viruses. Inflammatory exudates within the alveolar spaces lead to consolidation of the lung parenchyma, which results in dyspnea, tachypnea, and rales. Decreased vesicular breath sounds, dullness to percussion, and increased fremitus will be found over areas of consolidation.

191. The answer is D. *(Isselbacher, 13/e, pp 1197, 1206.)* Owing to destruction of alveolar septa in this patient, there is reduced elastic recoil, which may allow for collapse of the small airways and thereby prolong the expiratory phase of respiration. During this prolonged expiratory phase, the patient will characteristically be exhaling through "pursed lips" to avoid collapse of these small airways. The respiratory rate is increased by having a markedly shortened inspiratory interval. The patient may also be thin and asthenic, have an increased anteroposterior chest diameter, and evidence hypertrophy of the accessory muscles of respiration. The diaphragm may be depressed, and percussion will be hyperresonant.

192. The answer is C. *(Isselbacher, 13/e, pp 1214–1220.)* Most often the only symptom of pulmonary thromboembolism (PTE or PE) is sudden onset of unexplained dyspnea. Pleuritic chest pain and hemoptysis will only be present if pulmonic infarction has occurred. The most reliable symptom, however, is breathlessness. If the dyspnea is severe and persistent, this is an ominous sign because it usually indicates extensive embolic occlusion. An excellent clue to the diagnosis of PTE is deep venous thrombosis (DVT), but absence of signs and symptoms of DVT does not exclude PTE. Tachycardia is a single consistent sign. Common settings for the appearance of pulmonary embolism include prolonged immobilization, recent surgery, congestive heart failure, recent trauma (especially to the lower extremities), previous history of thrombophlebitis, use of oral contraceptives with a high estrogen content, sickle cell anemia, polycythemias, and inherited deficiencies of the anticoagulating proteins (antithrombin III, protein C).

193. The answer is D. *(Isselbacher, 13/e, pp 1163, 1186.)* The signs and symptoms of a lung abscess often include a history of alcoholism or intravenous drug abuse. There may be a latent period of several days or weeks during which only fever and malaise are noted. Cough, pleuritic pain, chills, and fever occur as the process develops. Within a few days the patient may suddenly cough up a large amount of foul-smelling, purulent sputum, usually blood-streaked or frankly bloody. Copious, malodorous sputum associated with the debility of long-standing infection is typical of chronic abscess.

194. The answer is C. *(Isselbacher, 13/e, pp 1206–1209.)* Idiopathic pulmonary fibrosis (IPF), also called the Hamman-Rich syndrome, is almost as common as sarcoidosis and occurs a little more commonly in males. Its peak occurrence is in the fifth and sixth decades of life. IPF usually presents first as exertional dyspnea, with or without a cough. X-ray films usually show evidence of fibrosis.

195. The answer is D. *(Isselbacher, 13/e, pp 1197–1206.)* Centrilobular emphysema involves, in its early stages, the proximal acini, which are the respiratory bronchioles, and thus has early sparing of the more distal air spaces. This disease is most commonly associated with cigarette smoking, and the patient will most often complain of steadily increasing dyspnea. A genetic deficiency of α_1-antitrypsin (a protease inhibitor) is associated with panacinar emphysema. A chest x-ray will show increased lung volume due to air trapping secondary to loss of elastic recoil. Because of this increased volume, the lungs are continuously in the inspiratory position, which gives rise to an increased anteroposterior diameter ("barrel chest").

196. The answer is C. *(Badgett, Am J Med 94:188, 1993.)* A recent study evaluated the best clinical predictors of chronic obstructive pulmonary disease (COPD). Two significant historical variables were found: history of smoking (70 or more pack-years) and prior diagnosis of COPD. The only physical sign that added significantly to the historical information was diminished breath sounds. A diminished peak flow on a flowmeter is also of some value in diagnosing COPD.

197. The answer is E. *(Isselbacher, 13/e, pp 1240–1243.)* Adult respiratory distress syndrome (ARDS) can occur as a consequence of conditions unrelated to direct pulmonary trauma, for example, burns, transfusion, or bodily trauma. ARDS is due to severe and widespread increased alveolar capillary permeability, secondary to injury of the alveolar lining epithelium and capillary endothelium. This leads to accumulation of a protein-rich edematous fluid within the septal walls, followed by escape of the fluid into the alveolar spaces, where it coagulates to form hyaline membranes lining the alveoli. As a consequence of the above, there is marked impairment of gas exchange, which causes severe dyspnea, wet rales, tachypnea, marked hypoxemia with cyanosis (which may be refractory to oxygen therapy), and diffuse bilateral pulmonary infiltrates on radiograph. Intensive medical care is necessary for this condition.

198. The answer is B. *(Isselbacher, 13/e, pp 1214–1220.)* Pulmonary embolism is the sole cause of death in about 100,000 patients per year in the U.S., and a contributory cause of death in an equal number of patients. In the U.S., it is the number three killer, preceded only by heart disease and cancer.

Occlusions of the pulmonary arteries by blood clots are almost always embolic; these emboli arise from thrombi in the deep veins of the legs. Secondary thrombosis may then build up around the emboli. Prolonged bed rest, immobilization of an extremity, congestive heart failure, burns, multiple fractures and any form of severe trauma, parturition, disseminated cancer, and use of oral contraceptives with high levels of estrogen are all common causes of pulmonary embolism. Sudden death from massive pulmonary embolism occurs when the blood supply of four out of the five pulmonary lobes becomes occluded. When there is occlusion to a branch of the pulmonary artery, radiolabeled albumin will not reach the lung distal to the blockage; thus, this area will show up as a "cold" area on a scan.

199. The answer is B. *(Seidel, 3/e, pp 340–341.)* Vesicular breath sounds are low-pitched and of low intensity and are sometimes described as "breezy." They are heard over the lesser bronchi, bronchioles, and lobes. Bronchovesicular breath sounds are normally heard over the main bronchi and are a combination of sounds made from normal vesicular breath sounds and bronchial breath sounds. They are likened to "air passing through a tube" and are highest in pitch and intensity. Vesicular breath sounds are normally heard over the apices of the lungs. Both bronchovesicular and bronchial breath sounds are abnormal if heard over the peripheral lung tissue. When the patient is upright, the uppermost portions of the lungs are the first to be inflated; thus, early maximal intensity occurs in the apices. The basilar portions of the lung have their maximal intensity later in the inspiratory cycle.

200. The answer is C. *(Seidel, 3/e, pp 340–346.)* Egophony is characterized by increased intensity of the spoken word upon auscultation. Whispered pectoriloquy occurs in areas of consolidation of the lung tissue; even a whisper can be heard clearly through a stethoscope. Vocal resonance is decreased when there is the opposite of consolidation, as appears in emphysema. Tympany to percussion occurs when there is increased air in the lungs or other air-filled viscera (e.g., the stomach); this represents the opposite of consolidation. When large accumulations of fluid press against the lower lung, voice sounds have a nasal quality over the upper lung. This is similar to skodaic resonance or percussion. Skodaic resonance is a unique, high-pitched sound, less musical than that of resonance obtained over a cavity; it is elicited by percussion just above a pleural effusion.

201. The answer is B. *(Seidel, 3/e, p 363.)* Croup results from a variety of viral agents, but most often from the parainfluenza viruses. Occurrence is most frequent in children between the ages of 1 and 3 years, and boys are more frequently affected. The inflammation is subglottic. The child usually awakens suddenly and is often very frightened. The cough is somewhat like the bark of a seal, and there is labored breathing, intercostal retractions, inspiratory stridor, and the use of accessory muscles of respiration.

202. The answer is D. *(Isselbacher, 13/e, p 519. Seidel, 3/e, p 364.)* Epiglottitis is an acute, life-threatening disease almost always caused by *Haemophilus influenzae* type b. Onset is sudden, and progression is rapid and often leads to full obstruction of the upper airway and a fatal outcome. It occurs most often in children between the ages of 3 and 7. The diagnosis can be established by a soft-tissue x-ray of the lateral neck that demonstrates the "thumb-print" sign of a swollen epiglottis. Examination with the aid of a tongue-blade should not be attempted unless preparations are made for possible tracheostomy because of the possibility that a laryngospasm may occur and occlude the airway totally.

203. The answer is D. *(Seidel, 3/e, pp 665, 669.)* In kyphosis there is pronounced dorsal curvature of the thoracic spine with flattening of the lumbar curvature. Pregnant women experience both structural and ventilatory changes. The costal angle is normally 68°, but in the third trimester it can increase up to 103°. Breathing becomes more thoracic than abdominal. The rate increases slightly by about 2 breaths per minute, and each breath is deeper. Infants normally have a rounded, or barrel, chest, and if this persists past the second year of life, the physician must examine for a chronic obstructive pulmonary disease such as cystic fibrosis. Inspection of the patient, including watching respiratory movement and effort, should be well under way by the time that the physical examination is begun.

204. The answer is D. *(Seidel, 3/e, pp 314–338.)* Posteriorly, the apices of the lungs rise to the level of T1. Upon forced expiration the lower borders of the lungs rise to the level of T10. These landmarks will vary when the patient has physical changes, such as obesity and chronic obstructive pulmonary disease. The trachea is a midline structure.

205. The answer is A. *(Isselbacher, 13/e, p 1232.)* In a tension pneumothorax, air enters the thorax on inspiration and becomes trapped upon expiration. This continuous process of leaking into the pleural space causes the ipsilateral lung to become compressed. As the collection of air increases, the breath sounds become faint because of the reduced inflation of the ipsilateral lung, and the percussion note will be tympanic in nature. In the late stages of this process, the greatly expanded pleural space will compress the contralateral pleural space and its associated lung. This process may push the trachea toward the uninvolved side. A spontaneous pneumothorax is more likely to occur in tall, thin, young persons. When the trachea is deviated away from the involved side, it is considered a medical emergency. Moderate-sized pneumothoraces can be aspirated with catheters that have one-way valves that allow air to escape and not to reenter. Most pneumothoraces are treated with closed thoracostomy tube drainage.

206. The answer is C. *(Isselbacher, 13/e, pp 2433–2437.)* Some of the more common adverse effects of smoking are cancers of the lung, COPD (chronic bronchitis and emphysema), myocardial infarction, and systemic atherosclerosis. Some of the less common adverse effects of cigarette smoking are peptic ulcer and cancer of the larynx, esophagus, kidney, pancreas, and bladder. There is no known association between cigarette smoking and ectopic pregnancy.

207. The answer is D. *(Isselbacher, 13/e, p 1232. Seidel, 3/e, p 360.)* With a penetrating wound to the thorax and deviation of the trachea away from the involved side, the physician can assume tension pneumothorax. Breath sounds will be distant, the percussion note will be hyperresonant, and fremitus will be decreased. There will not be rales or rhonchi on the affected side because the lung will be collapsed. The increased air on the affected side is in the pleural space, not in the lung. As an attempt is made to inflate the lung, air moves into the pleural space from the puncture site. This results in a collapsed lung with a large pleural space.

208. The answer is D. *(Isselbacher, 13/e, pp 1184–1191. Seidel, 3/e, pp 358–359.)* Pneumonia can be caused by a virus, bacteria, or mycoplasma and is characteristically accompanied by a cough with sputum production (productive cough), fever, chills, and pleuritic chest pain, all of which may have been preceded by an upper respiratory tract infection. Physical examination will uncover the many signs of consolidation of the lung parenchyma, including increased tactile and vocal fremitus, bronchophony, egophony, bronchial breath sounds, and possibly fine rales over the consolidated area. When there is also an associated pleural effusion, the examiner may find some contrary features, such as distant-to-absent breath sounds, a pleural friction rub (which may disappear as the effusion becomes significant), decreased fremitus, and flatness to percussion. The above signs are most often found with bacterial pneumonias, while the viral and mycoplasmal pneumonias characteristically show very few signs (often only rales are heard).

209. The answer is C. *(Isselbacher, 13/e, p 1173.)* With inhalation of noxious gas, the patient will usually have conjunctivitis, pharyngitis, wheezing, and acute bronchitis. Since phosgene does not irritate the upper airways, it can be inhaled in sufficient concentrations to produce pulmonary congestion and edema, without irritation of the epiglottis. Phosgene, like other poisonous gases, may cause nausea and dizziness.

210. The answer is C. *(Isselbacher, 13/e, pp 998–1009.)* Congestive heart failure (CHF) has the pulmonary manifestation known as cardiogenic pulmonary edema. There is most often a history of hypertension or heart disease. Cardiomegaly is suggested when there is lateral and downward displacement of the apical impulse. A summation gallop is due to the occurrence of the third and fourth heart sounds together, which results from an increased heart rate and decreased diastolic time. Most patients with CHF will have increased heart rate, and thus a summation gallop may be found. Murmurs may be present. Fine, moist, basilar rales and wheezing (cardiac asthma) may be evident.

211. The answer is E. *(Seidel, 3/e, p 330.)* Pectus excavatum (funnel breast) is a congenital, hereditary malformation characterized by depression of the sternum below the clavicular-manubrial junction with symmetric inward bending of the costal cartilages. As the infant develops, kyphosis may occur. Severe degrees of funnel breast may embarrass pulmonary and cardiac function. Pectus excavatum is not associated with other midline defects, such as cleft palate.

212. The answer is C. *(Seidel, 3/e, pp 353–354.)* If pleural effusion develops, pleuritic pain and the friction rub lessen, tactile fremitus to the spoken voice diminishes, and there is dullness to percussion. Breath sounds may be exaggerated or bronchial in the area of effusion; however, breath sounds are usually decreased in association with a pleural effusion. Similarly, egophony is decreased.

213. The answer is B. *(Isselbacher, 13/e, pp 1167–1172.)* Asthma is an airway disease that is characterized by a hyperreactive tracheobronchial tree that manifests physiologically as narrowing of the air passages. The classic triad of symptoms seen in asthma is dyspnea, cough, and wheezing, with the last being the *sine qua non.* In its most typical form, asthma is an episodic disease and attacks occur most often at night, perhaps due to circadian variations in the circulating levels of endogenous catecholamines and histamine. Attacks may also occur abruptly following exposure to a specific allergen, physical exertion, a viral respiratory infection, or emotional excitement. At the onset the patient will sense a constriction about the chest, often with a nonproductive cough. Respiration will become harsh, and wheezing in both phases of respiration will develop. The expiratory phase will become prolonged, and the patient frequently will have tachypnea, tachycardia, and mild systolic hypertension. If the attack is severe or prolonged, the accessory muscles of respiration will be visibly active and frequently a pulsus paradoxus will develop. These two signs correlate well with the degree of obstruction and the probability of hospitalization.

214. The answer is B. *(Isselbacher, 13/e, pp 519, 653.)* Acute epiglottitis is a progressive cellulitis of the epiglottis and surrounding tissues in the supraglottic airway that can cause acute airway obstruction. In young patients the causative organism is most frequently *Haemophilus influenzae* type b. In adolescents and adults the epiglottitis may not be as fulminant, and the most common organisms isolated in these cases are *Streptococcus pneumoniae* and *Staphylococcus aureus.* Frequent complaints include dysphagia, odynophagia, and a fever that has progressed over 1 to 2 days. Stridor may be present, but hoarseness and loss of voice power are nearly universal. The patient will prefer to lean forward, and drooling may be seen. An edematous, cherry-red epiglottis and surrounding pharyngeal mucosa will be seen upon examination, and this visualization is the best way to confirm the diagnosis in adults. Examination of the pharynx is contraindicated in children because of the risk of laryngospasm and the resultant airway obstruction. In children a lateral x-ray of the neck will show an enlarged epiglottis, the "thumbprint" sign.

215. The answer is C. *(Isselbacher, 13/e, pp 519, 806.)* Laryngotracheobronchitis (LTB), or croup, is a syndrome produced by acute infection of the lower air passages and most commonly occurs in children 3 years old or younger. The most common causative agent is the parainfluenza virus, but a wide variety of respiratory viruses and *Mycoplasma pneumoniae* can also cause LTB. The clinical hallmark is a barking or brassy cough. The epiglottis is not involved, and croup can easily be distinguished from epiglottitis by examination of a lateral neck x-ray, which will show no epiglottal edema. Management of LTB requires hospitalization, close observation, humidification, and oxygenation as directed by pulse oximetry. Only rarely will intubation be necessary.

216. The answer is D. *(Isselbacher, 13/e, pp 1194–1197.)* This is a typical clinical presentation of cystic fibrosis. There is nearly always a history of recurrent respiratory infections (90 percent) with a persistent cough between attacks and failure to thrive (85 percent). A history of meconium ileus occurs in 5 percent of cases. The most common organisms responsible for the respiratory infections are *Staphylococcus aureus* and *Pseudomonas aeruginosa,* both of which produce the large amounts of mucus that cause the earliest obstructive lesions in the bronchi and bronchioles.

217. The answer is A. *(Isselbacher, 13/e, pp 2037–2039.)* Gynecomastia is seen in about 55 to 60 percent of adolescent boys and usually occurs during Tanner stage 2 or 3. It is usually painful and may be unilateral or bilateral. It gradually appears and it gradually disappears within 1 year of onset. Pubertal changes that occur during Tanner stages 2 and 3 include growth spurt, growth of testes and penis, spermarche, acne, axillary perspiration, and appearance of pubic hair. You can reassure the boy and ask that he come back monthly. If the gynecomastia does not resolve, it will be necessary to rule out Klinefelter's syndrome (which has obvious signs), adrenal tumors, gonadal tumors, hypothyroidism, hepatic disorders, and use of drugs, especially marijuana.

218. The answer is C. *(Isselbacher, 13/e, pp 1167–1172, 1537, 2223–2233.)* Asthma is episodic with most exacerbations at night, but it can also commonly occur in response to a specific allergen, physical exertion, a viral respiratory infection, or emotional excitement. Foreign body obstruction almost always presents with inspiratory stridor, and the harsh respiratory sounds can be localized to the trachea or an individual bronchus. Epilepsy would present with a characteristic seizure and postictal event and does not present solely as a respiratory distress situation. Carcinoid tumors can cause recurrent episodes of bronchospasm, but this patient's history of taking medication along with the rarity of these tumors leads the physician to diagnose the more common asthma. Chronic bronchitis can cause recurrent episodes of bronchospasm, but with this disease there are no true symptom-free periods and patients are typically older smokers.

219. The answer is B. *(Behrman, 15/e, p 550.)* In choanal atresia, the baby looks fine when crying but turns blue when crying stops. It is necessary to maintain the airway, and one way to do this temporarily is to make a large hole in the pacifier. The incidence of unilateral choanal atresia is 1:2500 live births; bilateral choanal atresia occurs in 1:5000 live births. The latter condition warrants immediate surgical correction.

220. The answer is D. *(Seidel, 3/e, pp 349–364.)* In the pediatric population, croup and epiglottitis are two diseases that present with stridor, but the differential diagnosis must include laryngotracheal bronchitis, bacterial tracheitis, diphtheria, measles, vocal cord paralysis, congenital laryngeal stridor, congenital airway webs, congenital airway stenosis, foreign body aspiration, intrinsic mass, and extrinsic tracheal compression by mass or enlarged aberrant vessels. When there is extrathoracic obstruction, the inspiratory obstruction is greater than the expiratory obstruction. When there is intrathoracic obstruction, the expiratory obstruction is greater than the inspiratory obstruction. Infants have an increased susceptibility to upper airway obstruction.

221. The answer is C. *(Markovchick, p 10.)* By far, the tongue is the most common cause of airway obstruction. With a decreased level of consciousness there is decreased muscle tone and the tongue falls posteriorly to obstruct the oropharynx. The quickest method to correct this situation is the head tilt/chin lift maneuver.

222. The answer is B. *(Isselbacher, 13/e, pp 761–762.)* This clinical presentation is fairly typical of chlamydial pneumonia. The history of a prior mild conjunctivitis that responded to erythromycin also lends support to a diagnosis of chlamydial infection. Most chlamydial pneumonias will present between the ages of 3 and 11 weeks, and most will present after 1 week of persistent symptoms. The majority will manifest a staccato cough with bilateral rales. This could represent a mild case of pertussis, but in the unimmunized infant pertussis is unlikely to be mild in appearance. An absolute eosinophil count of greater than 400 correlates well with chlamydial pneumonia, whereas you would most likely see a lymphocytosis with pertussis. There are now enzyme-linked immunoassays that can be used on nasopharyngeal specimens, or chlamydial inclusion bodies can be seen with Wright's or Giemsa's stains. Topical erythromycin will eradicate the conjunctivitis, but it will not eradicate the nasopharyngeal carrier state that has been established; therefore, it is now recommended that oral erythromycin be administered at 40 mg per kilogram body weight per day in four doses for 14 days. A bacterial pneumonia, such as group B streptococcal pneumonia, would present more acutely and the patient would appear very ill. Respiratory syncytial viral (RSV) pneumonia appears very much like chlamydial pneumonia, but with this past history of conjunctivitis it is not the most likely diagnosis. Aspiration pneumonia usually does not occur in the healthy child, and when it occurs the chest roentgenograph will usually reveal an alveolar infiltrate.

223. The answer is A. *(Markovchick, pp 9–10.)* The first vital sign to change in the face of respiratory distress is the respiratory rate. Diaphoresis, along with somnolence, are signs of hypercapnia and respiratory acidosis. Restlessness and cyanosis are seen with hypoxia. Vigorous use of accessory muscles is an ominous sign and needs immediate attention. Pursed-lip breathing is most often a learned behavior that occurs with emphysema; it is done to prolong the expiratory phase of respiration and prevent sudden collapse of small airways.

224. The answer is B. *(Isselbacher, 13/e, pp 1192, 2013.)* Kartagener's syndrome belongs to a group of inheritable disorders known as *immotile cilia syndromes.* Kartagener's syndrome is known by the triad of dextrocardia (or situs inversus), chronic sinusitis (with formation of nasal polyps), and bronchiectasis. There is a defect that causes the cilia within the respiratory tract epithelium to be immotile, as well as the cilia of sperm.

225. The answer is E. *(Isselbacher, 13/e, pp 787–790.)* Shingles is a disease that usually occurs many years after an initial infection of chickenpox, which is caused by herpes zoster. For unknown reasons, the virus, which had been latent in the nerve, reactivates and expresses itself along the dermatome. The painful dermatomic lesions begin as erythema then progress to vesicular and pustular eruptions, which burst and crust over. Open wounds are contagious. The pain appears to be worse in the elderly and immunocompromised.

226. The answer is A. *(Isselbacher, 13/e, pp 148, 150, 1197–1206.)* COPD is characterized by hyperinflated lungs that are secondary to destruction of lung parenchyma and lead to an increase in anteroposterior diameter of the chest ("barrel chest"), hyperresonance, and decreased tactile fremitus. Stridor is a high-pitched sound heard on inspiration that suggests obstruction in the upper respiratory tree. Biot's respiration is an irregular pattern of breathing usually associated with a significant increase in intracranial pressure.

227–231. The answers are 227-B, 228-D, 229-C, 230-A, 231-E. *(Isselbacher, 13/e, pp 1103, 1233, 1362, 1442, 1908.)* Routine posteroanterior and lateral chest films are very helpful in diseases of the chest in that they help to localize masses. The appearance of the mass and its mediastinal location often lead to a correct diagnosis. When a patient presents with symptoms of myasthenia gravis and a lateral chest x-ray reveals an anterior calcified mass, the tumor is almost always a thymoma. A teratoma can have tissue derived from all three embryonic layers, and a tooth would be virtually diagnostic. Two views, as always, are necessary because an aspirated tooth may give the novice observer the appearance of a teratoma. Phlebolith suggests a hemangioma. Gas detected in the mediastinum could indicate a hiatal hernia, a ruptured esophagus, or a pneumomediastinum. When a radiologist uses the term *grade 5 density*, this indicates the presence of a foreign object.

232–236. The answers are 232-C, 233-A, 234-B, 235-D, 236-E. *(Berkow, 16/e, p 602. Seidel, 3/e, pp 331–332, 340–341.)* Cheyne-Stokes respiration has a regular periodic pattern of breathing, with intervals of apnea followed by a crescendo/decrescendo sequence of respiration. It is also known as *periodic breathing.* Children and older adults may breathe in this pattern during sleep, but otherwise it occurs only in patients who are seriously ill, often with cardiogenic or neurogenic problems. In heart failure, slowing of the circulation is the predominant cause; a combination of acidosis and hypoxia in the respiratory centers can also contribute significantly.

Kussmaul's breathing is a distinctive pattern of slow, deep respirations and is commonly induced by diabetic acidosis (blood pH 7.2 or lower). The breathing capacity is maintained; thus, the patient rarely complains of dyspnea.

Biot's respiration is characterized by intense and noisy hyperventilation of 4 to 5 breaths of similar depth with unpredictably irregular periods of apnea. Biot's respiration is most often associated with persistent and severe increased intracranial pressure and is often the result of a cerebral lesion, such as hemorrhage.

Hyperventilation is often confused with tachypnea, which is simply a persistent respiratory rate in excess of 20 breaths per minute. Hyperventilation is tachypnea coupled with hyperpnea (deep respirations). Central nervous system disease, metabolic disease (such as hepatic encephalopathy), exercise, and anxiety can all cause hyperpnea.

Rapid, shallow breathing with prolonged expiration can result from emphysema. Owing to reduced elastic recoil, the patient must breathe more often because the depth of respiration is reduced.

237–241. The answers are 237-E, 238-A, 239-D, 240-C, 241-B. *(Seidel, 3/e, pp 450–468.)* If a woman under the age of 30 presents with a mobile mass that has well-defined borders, it is most likely a fibroadenoma, which is a benign condition; however, breast cancer must be ruled out.

In 70 to 80 percent of patients who seek professional consultation for a breast mass, the mass is hard and well circumscribed. When it is also fixed to the skin or a deep muscle, or if there is edema or retraction of the nipple, it is almost certainly carcinoma of the breast. Most breast carcinomas present in the upper outer quadrant of the breast.

Intraductal papilloma can present with a bloody nipple discharge, which is a classic sign of cancer. This tumor is benign, however, and does not present with a palpable mass.

Characteristics of inflammatory breast carcinoma include increased local temperature, redness, and an erysipeloid margin, and the entire breast is usually indurated and firm-to-hard. The prognosis is very poor because most often at the time of presentation the tumor has widely metastasized.

Paget's disease classically presents with eczematoid changes in the nipple, including itching, burning, oozing, and bleeding, which all occur over a relatively long period of time. A mass can be palpated in up to two-thirds of these patients.

242–244. The answers are 242-A, 243-A, 244-C. *(Isselbacher, 13/e, pp 1184–1191.)* Viral pneumonia accounts for approximately 90 percent of pneumonias in children. A predisposing factor in viral pneumonia is illness in other family members. Symptoms include cough, fever, chills, sweating, and bradycardia. Onset is gradual, the course is mild, sputum is minimal, and there may be few rales, which are bilateral and diffuse.

Bacterial pneumonia accounts for approximately 10 percent of pneumonias in children. There is usually a minor upper respiratory infection prior to onset, which is abrupt. The disease is severe, and presentation often includes high fever, cough, dyspnea, tachycardia, rusty sputum, consolidation of lung parenchyma, neutrophilia, positive sputum culture, and positive blood culture.

245–249. The answers are 245-B, 246-B, 247-A, 248-A, 249-A. *(Isselbacher, 13/e, pp 519, 806. Seidel, 3/e, p 363.)* Epiglottitis is a serious infection caused almost invariably by *Haemophilus influenzae* and most common during the ages of 3 to 7 years. Epiglottitis does not have a seasonal preference. The patient will complain of a very sore throat and dysphagia and will often be drooling from the mouth. A fever usually greater than 39.44°C (103°F) and leukocytosis with a left shift will be present. On a lateral soft-tissue x-ray of the neck, one will see the classic "thumb-print" sign, which represents a swollen epiglottis. When epiglottitis is strongly suspected, you should not attempt to examine the epiglottis unless you are adequately prepared for a difficult intubation secondary to the laryngospasm that may ensue.

Viral croup occurs most commonly in the fall and winter, and most often in the age group of 3 months to 3 years. The most common etiologic agent is parainfluenza virus. There will usually be a several-day history of a coryza-like prodrome, with or without a sore throat. The temperature will usually be less than 39.44°C (103°F) and the total white blood cell count will usually be normal. The diagnosis is made by clinical presentation and is one of exclusion. Diagnosis can be aided with an anteroposterior x-ray of the larynx, which will show subglottic narrowing, known as the "steeple sign."

Abdomen

DIRECTIONS: Each item below contains a question or incomplete statement followed by suggested responses. Select the **one best** response to each question.

250. The proper sequence for examination of the abdomen is

(A) auscultation, percussion, inspection, palpation
(B) auscultation, inspection, palpation, percussion
(C) inspection, auscultation, percussion, palpation
(D) inspection, percussion, palpation, auscultation
(E) none of the above

251. Indications of biliary obstruction include all the following EXCEPT

(A) black, tarry stools
(B) jaundice
(C) scleral icterus
(D) dark urine
(E) pruritus

252. All the following are signs of ascites EXCEPT

(A) bulging flanks
(B) puddle sign
(C) fluid wave
(D) shifting dullness
(E) purple striae

253. A 68-year-old man presents with a chief complaint that solid food gets stuck in the middle of his chest. In addition, he admits to a 25-pound weight loss over the last 3 months. The most likely diagnosis is

(A) esophagitis
(B) lower esophageal ring
(C) esophageal carcinoma
(D) cerebrovascular accident
(E) myocardial infarction

254. A 55-year-old man presents to the hospital with the complaint of severe intermittent pain in his right lower back that radiates around his trunk into his lower quadrant and upper right thigh. The most likely diagnosis is

(A) hepatitis
(B) appendicitis
(C) a ureteral stone
(D) pyelonephritis
(E) biliary obstruction

255. Signs and symptoms consistent with acute appendicitis include all the following EXCEPT

(A)   diffuse periumbilical pain
(B)   fever greater than 40°C (104°F)
(C)   nausea and vomiting
(D)   pain in the right lower quadrant
(E)   rebound tenderness

256. A 38-year-old woman who presents with a history of sudden chills, fever, abdominal pain, backache, nausea, and vomiting is found to have costovertebral angle tenderness, with erythrocytes and WBCs in her urine. The most likely diagnosis is

(A)   cholangitis
(B)   cystitis
(C)   cholecystitis
(D)   pyelonephritis
(E)   pancreatitis

257. All the following are true of abdominal striae EXCEPT

(A)   they are transverse marks on the abdominal wall
(B)   they may be associated with pregnancy
(C)   they may be associated with Cushing's syndrome
(D)   they may be associated with rapid gain and loss of weight
(E)   they may be red or purple

258. Which of the following statements is true of examination of the abdomen?

(A)   The quadrant of maximal pain should be carefully examined first
(B)   The hips and knees should be extended throughout the examination
(C)   After palpation, percussion and auscultation should be performed
(D)   Auscultation should be terminated if no bowel sounds are heard within 1 min
(E)   There should always be hepatic dullness to percussion in the right midaxillary line

259. A 42-year-old woman presents to the emergency room complaining of abdominal pain. While you are palpating under her right costal margin, she abruptly arrests her inspiration and pulls away because of sharp pain. The most likely diagnosis at this time is

(A)   pulmonary embolism
(B)   acute pancreatitis
(C)   alcoholic cirrhosis
(D)   acute gastritis
(E)   acute cholecystitis

260. McBurney's point is located

(A) in the midclavicular line just under the right costal margin

(B) at the midpoint of a line connecting the symphysis pubis and the anterior superior iliac spine

(C) midway along the right inguinal ligament

(D) one-third of the way along a line drawn from the right anterior superior iliac spine to the umbilicus

(E) at the point of maximum tenderness in a patient with acute pancreatitis

261. A 16-year-old boy presents in the emergency room with a history of a football injury to the left flank earlier that day. He reports that at the time of injury he only had the wind knocked out of him and recovered in a few minutes. About 1 h later he began to experience pain in the left upper quadrant and left shoulder and light-headedness on standing. The diagnosis that would best explain these symptoms is

(A) dislocation of the left shoulder

(B) broken rib on the left side

(C) collapsed lung

(D) contusion of the left kidney

(E) ruptured spleen

262. All the following statements about physical findings in a patient with peritonitis are true EXCEPT

(A) in extreme cases, abdominal rigidity (guarding) results in persistent abdominal wall stiffness, which prevents movement of the abdomen during inspiration

(B) the abdominal wall may be flaccid

(C) having the patient lift the head so that the chin touches the chest will worsen the tenderness elicited on abdominal palpation

(D) rebound tenderness results from the passive movement of the abdominal wall to its pretested position

(E) the referred rebound test is performed at an area away from the area of tenderness and results in pain in the area of maximal tenderness

263. All the following are signs of portal hypertension EXCEPT

(A) caput medusae

(B) hemorrhoids

(C) esophageal varices

(D) papilledena

(E) spider angiomata

264. A characteristic of femoral hernias is that

(A) they result from a weakness in Hesselbach's triangle
(B) they are the same as an indirect inguinal hernia
(C) they present about 2 cm medial to the femoral artery
(D) unlike other inguinal hernias, they are not associated with increased intraabdominal pressure
(E) they are more common in males

265. A 71-year-old woman with a history of coronary artery disease presents to her family physician for a routine check-up. The physician notices that she has lost 20 pounds since her last visit 6 months ago. When questioned, she gives a history of intermittent periumbilical pain that always begins about 30 min after eating and lasts about 2 h. She claims that the pain is worse after large meals and so she has begun to eat less out of fear of the pain. The most likely diagnosis is

(A) pancreatitis
(B) cholecystitis
(C) small bowel obstruction
(D) intestinal ischemia
(E) peptic ulcer disease

266. All the following statements concerning inguinal hernias are correct EXCEPT

(A) a hernia through the posterior wall of the inguinal canal is termed *indirect*
(B) the site of the bulge of a direct inguinal hernia is medial to that of an indirect inguinal hernia
(C) the indirect inguinal hernia is the most common of all abdominal hernias
(D) in either sex, a small indirect hernia may produce a bulge over the midpoint of the inguinal ligament
(E) finding an indirect hernia on one side increases the likelihood of finding an indirect hernia on the opposite side

267. All the following conditions are usually associated with the finding of decreased bowel sounds EXCEPT

(A) advanced intestinal obstruction
(B) peritonitis
(C) mesenteric thrombosis
(D) brisk diarrhea
(E) ileus

268. All the following are signs of peritoneal irritation EXCEPT

(A) rebound tenderness (Blumberg's sign)
(B) tenderness to light percussion of the abdomen
(C) jar tenderness (Markel's sign)
(D) voluntary rigidity of abdominal musculature
(E) guarding

269. Which of the following statements is true of the scaphoid abdomen?

(A) An unremarkable abdomen should be recorded as "scaphoid"

(B) It is convex anteriorly

(C) It is seen in patients with severe ascites

(D) It would not be expected in an obese patient

(E) It implies guarding or rigidity

270. The span of the normal adult liver is

(A) 6 to 12 cm in the mid-clavicular line

(B) 12 to 16 cm in the mid-clavicular line

(C) 2 to 4 cm in the midsternal line

(D) undetectable in the midsternal line

(E) greater in women than men

271. A 48-year-old man with a history of alcohol abuse presents to the emergency room vomiting bright red blood. All the following should be included in the differential diagnosis EXCEPT

(A) ruptured esophageal varices

(B) esophageal reflux secondary to a hiatal hernia

(C) Boerhaave's syndrome

(D) Mallory-Weiss syndrome

(E) a bleeding peptic ulcer

272. If acute appendicitis progresses to perforation, all the following physical findings are likely to be seen EXCEPT

(A) a positive obturator test

(B) a positive Murphy's sign

(C) rebound tenderness (Blumberg's sign)

(D) jar tenderness (Markel's sign)

(E) a positive iliopsoas test

273. Epidemiologic studies show that cholelithiasis (gallstones) occurs more commonly in all the following groups of people EXCEPT

(A) pregnant women

(B) women taking estrogen

(C) obese people

(D) people greater than 60 years of age

(E) diabetics

274. An accurate characterization of jaundice is that it

(A) occurs when the serum bilirubin level exceeds 2 to 4 mg/dL

(B) may be noticed in the sclerae before it can be detected in the blood

(C) can be confused with scleral discoloration of carotene or quinacrine

(D) usually presents as a green discoloration of the skin

(E) is usually most intense in the extremities

275. Which of the following statements is true of the clinical diagnosis of acute appendicitis in patients more than 50 years of age?

(A) Clinical diagnosis is not reliable
(B) Pain is not a significant predictor
(C) Abdominal rigidity is not a significant predictor
(D) Tenderness is not a significant predictor
(E) Pain, rigidity, and tenderness are all significant predictors

276. A 42-year-old man presents with a history of burning epigastric pain that begins 1 to 4 h postprandially. He reports that this pain is relieved either by food or antacid tablets. The most likely diagnosis is

(A) cholecystitis
(B) acute pancreatitis
(C) a peptic ulcer
(D) intestinal angina
(E) celiac sprue

277. When a patient presents with a history of coffee-ground emesis and black, tarry stools, all the following are likely etiologies EXCEPT

(A) peptic ulcer
(B) diverticular hemorrhage
(C) gastritis
(D) duodenal ulcer
(E) esophageal varices

278. The stigmata of chronic liver disease include all the following EXCEPT

(A) spider angiomata
(B) gynecomastia
(C) testicular atrophy
(D) parotid atrophy
(E) jaundice

279. All the following statements about palpation of the liver are correct EXCEPT

(A) a stony, hard liver is usually due to tumor
(B) a very firm liver with a sharp, hard edge is usually cirrhotic
(C) hepatomegaly is evident when the liver is easily palpated at 6 cm below the right costal margin
(D) when hepatic nodules are found by palpation, they are usually due to cancer rather than nodular cirrhosis
(E) expansive systolic hepatic pulsations are frequently a sign of tricuspid insufficiency

280. Common findings in intestinal obstruction include all the following EXCEPT

(A) ascites
(B) distention
(C) vomiting
(D) abdominal pain
(E) constipation

281. All the following are true statements concerning the spleen EXCEPT

(A) patients with sickle cell disease commonly have splenomegaly

(B) the spleen, in contrast to other masses in the left upper quadrant, moves greatly with inspiration

(C) when an enlarged spleen is found to be hard upon palpation, this is usually due to a chronic process

(D) splenomegaly in a patient with jaundice may be associated with a hemolytic anemia

(E) massive splenomegaly is seen in patients with chronic granulocytic leukemia

282. While auscultating a patient's abdomen, the examiner hears a systolic bruit in the midepigastric area. It occurs at a fixed interval after the impulse palpated at the cardiac apex. The most likely source of this bruit is

(A) the hepatic artery
(B) the splenic artery
(C) the abdominal aorta
(D) one of the renal arteries
(E) a transmitted heart murmur

283. All the following symptoms are common features of renal cell carcinoma EXCEPT

(A) gross hematuria
(B) flank pain
(C) palpable abdominal mass
(D) fatigability
(E) hypocalcemia

284. True statements concerning colon cancer include all the following EXCEPT

(A) lesions of the left colon commonly ulcerate and lead to chronic, insidious blood loss

(B) lesions of the right colon usually do not change the appearance of the stool

(C) tumors arising in the descending colon present with abdominal cramping, occasional obstruction, and even perforation

(D) neoplasms arising in the rectosigmoid often are associated with hematochezia, tenesmus, and a reduction in the caliber of the stool

(E) patients with tumors of the ascending colon commonly present with fatigue

285. True statements about abdominal aortic aneurysms include all the following EXCEPT

(A) they are most commonly found in patients with atherosclerosis

(B) frequently patients present with low or middle back pain

(C) on physical examination the aneurysm presents as an expansile, pulsating mass palpable between the umbilicus and xiphoid process

(D) the mass cannot be moved cephalad or caudad

(E) in 90 percent of cases a bruit can be heard over the aneurysm

DIRECTIONS: Each group of questions below consists of lettered options followed by numbered items. For each numbered item, select the appropriate lettered option(s). Each lettered option may be used once, more than once, or not at all. **Choose exactly the number of options indicated following each item.**

Items 286–289

Match the percussed sound with the organ over which the sound would occur.

(A) Liver
(B) Stomach
(C) Emphysematous lung
(D) Normal lung

286. Tympany **(SELECT 1 ORGAN)**

287. Hyperresonance **(SELECT 1 ORGAN)**

288. Resonance **(SELECT 1 ORGAN)**

289. Dullness **(SELECT 1 ORGAN)**

Items 290–293

Match the characteristics of pain below with the most probable condition.

(A) Infection
(B) Peptic ulcer
(C) Intestinal obstruction
(D) Pancreatitis

290. Burning **(SELECT 1 CONDITION)**

291. Cramping **(SELECT 1 CONDITION)**

292. Knifelike **(SELECT 1 CONDITION)**

293. Gradual onset **(SELECT 1 CONDITION)**

Items 294–298

Match the conditions below with the abdominal region where the associated pain is most commonly perceived.

(A) Right upper quadrant (RUQ)
(B) Right lower quadrant (RLQ)
(C) Periumbilical region
(D) Left upper quadrant (LUQ)
(E) Left lower quadrant (LLQ)

294. Early appendicitis **(SELECT 1 REGION)**

295. Meckel's diverticulitis **(SELECT 1 REGION)**

296. Sigmoid diverticulitis **(SELECT 1 REGION)**

297. Leaking duodenal ulcer **(SELECT 1 REGION)**

298. Ruptured spleen **(SELECT 1 REGION)**

Items 299–302

Match the most probable diagnosis with each patient.

(A) Perinephric abscess
(B) Peritonitis
(C) Intestinal obstruction
(D) Portal hypertension
(E) None of the above

299. A patient who remains motionless **(SELECT 1 DIAGNOSIS)**

300. A patient who is restless and moves about **(SELECT 1 DIAGNOSIS)**

301. A patient who rests with the trunk bent to the affected side **(SELECT 1 DIAGNOSIS)**

302. A patient with prominent, snakelike longitudinal veins passing from the inferior to superior aspect of the abdomen **(SELECT 1 DIAGNOSIS)**

Items 303–306

Match the signs and symptoms below with the most likely diagnosis.

(A) Cholangitis
(B) Pancreatic cancer
(C) Mesenteric artery occlusion
(D) Intussusception

303. Painless distention of the gallbladder (Courvoisier's sign) **(SELECT 1 DIAGNOSIS)**

304. Dance's sign **(SELECT 1 DIAGNOSIS)**

305. Abdominal pain out of proportion to physical findings **(SELECT 1 DIAGNOSIS)**

306. Abdominal pain, fever and chills, and jaundice (Charcot's triad) **(SELECT 1 DIAGNOSIS)**

Items 307–310

Match the causes of epigastric pain with the most likely temporal relationships.

(A) Early postprandial pain
(B) Pain at night and with recumbency
(C) Pain relieved by ingestion of food
(D) Late postprandial pain (several hours after eating)

307. Reflux esophagitis **(SELECT 1 PAIN)**

308. Gastric outlet obstruction **(SELECT 1 PAIN)**

309. Acute gastritis **(SELECT 1 PAIN)**

310. Duodenal ulcer **(SELECT 1 PAIN)**

DIRECTIONS: The group of questions below consists of four lettered options followed by a set of numbered items. For each numbered item select

A	if the item is associated with	(A) only
B	if the item is associated with	(B) only
C	if the item is associated with	**both** (A) and (B)
D	if the item is associated with	**neither** (A) nor (B)

Each lettered option may be used **once, more than once, or not at all.**

Items 311–316

(A) Ulcerative colitis
(B) Crohn's disease
(C) Both
(D) Neither

311. The major symptoms are bloody diarrhea and abdominal pain, often with fever and weight loss in more severe cases

312. The major clinical features are fever, abdominal pain, nonbloody diarrhea, and generalized fatigability

313. It is commonly the result of overgrowth of *Clostridium difficile* secondary to the use of antibiotics

314. Perirectal fistulas are not uncommon

315. The risk of developing a subsequent colonic malignancy is greatly increased

316. Physical examination often reveals tenderness of the right lower quadrant with an associated palpable mass that reflects adherent loops of bowel

Abdomen

Answers

250. The answer is C. *(Seidel, 3/e, pp 482–521, 787.)* It is necessary to auscultate the abdomen prior to percussion and palpation, as percussion may alter the frequency and intensity of bowel sounds. The absence of bowel sounds is not established unless no sounds are detected during 5 min of continuous auscultation. Percussion is an important means of assessing the size and density of abdominal organs, as well as of detecting fluid or air in the abdomen.

251. The answer is A. *(Isselbacher, 13/e, pp 1509–1512.)* Obstruction of the biliary tract prohibits bile from entering the intestine. When this occurs the stools are acholic and often malodorous with a white or gray color (clay-colored stools). Black, tarry stools (melena) are associated with gastrointestinal bleeding. Jaundice and scleral icterus result from conjugated bilirubin that builds up in the blood when it cannot pass through the biliary system. Jaundice usually appears at bilirubin levels of 2 to 4 mg/dL of serum. Since the bilirubin has already been conjugated by the liver, it is water-soluble and can be filtered into the urine, which turns dark. When bile salts build up in the skin, sensory nerves can be irritated, which causes intense pruritus that may become excruciating.

252. The answer is E. *(Cattau, JAMA 247:1164, 1982. Isselbacher, 13/e, pp 1960–1965.)* Purple striae are found in Cushing's syndrome. If distention from ascites causes striae, they will be pink or blue in early stages and silvery in late stages. Bulging flanks result from the weight of free fluid pushing the flanks outward. A fluid wave is a wave in the ascitic fluid elicited by tapping one side of the abdomen and felt by the receiving hand on the opposite side. This wave takes perceptible time to cross the abdomen. Fat in the mesentery may cause a similar wave, but it can be blocked by having the patient or an assistant press on the mid abdomen with the medial aspect of the hand. This maneuver does not block the fluid wave. *Shifting dullness* refers to the area of dullness in the dependent area of the abdomen. This area shifts with changes in body position.

253. The answer is C. *(Isselbacher, 13/e, pp 206–207, 1360–1382.)* Esophageal carcinoma occurs in the elderly with a history of weeks to months of progressive dysphagia associated with weight loss. In younger age groups, carcinoma of the bronchus and lymphomas can cause similar symptoms from enlarged perihilar lymph nodes that compress the esophagus.

254. The answer is C. *(Isselbacher, 13/e, pp 550, 1313–1334.)* Ureteral obstruction causes a severe colicky pain that often originates in the costovertebral angle and radiates around the trunk into the lower quadrant of the abdomen and possibly on into the upper thigh and testicle or labium. Vomiting is usually severe. Micturition may be painful and produce bloody urine.

255. The answer is B. *(Isselbacher, 13/e, pp 1433–1435.)* In acute appendicitis the normal progression of events is (1) diffuse periumbilical pain, (2) nausea and vomiting, (3) shifting of pain from epigastrium to right lower quadrant with the development of deep tenderness there, (4) fever (usually between 37.22 and 38.33°C [99 and 101°F]), and (5) leukocytosis (usually between 10,000 and 20,000 cells per microliter).

256. The answer is D. *(Isselbacher, 13/e, pp 548–553.)* Pyelonephritis is a bacterial infection of the kidney. Symptoms include sudden chills, fever, abdominal pain, backache, nausea, vomiting, and pain with urination. Signs include fever, costovertebral angle tenderness, enlarged and tender kidney, and abdominal muscle spasm. Urinalysis demonstrates leukocytes, erythrocytes, and bacteria.

257. The answer is A. *(Sapira, p 373.)* Abdominal striae are longitudinal stretch marks on the abdominal wall. They may be associated with pregnancy, Cushing's syndrome, and rapid gain and loss of weight. Striae are purple in cases of idiopathic Cushing's syndrome because of the erythrocytosis from the excess adrenal androgens. Other causes usually result in pink-red striae in the early stages.

258. The answer is E. *(Sapira, pp 373–377.)* All the quadrants of the abdomen should be examined in an orderly sequence. If the patient is complaining of pain, the order should be altered so that the painful area is examined last. Flexing the hips and knees with the soles of the feet in the bed will often help the patient relax the abdominal musculature. Auscultation of the abdomen should be performed before palpation or percussion. Palpation and percussion may disturb the peritoneal contents and silence the abdomen. The tinkles (sounds of musical timbre one or two octaves higher than normal) and rushes (sounds accelerated at least three times normal speed) of small bowel obstruction may occur 10 to 20 min apart. The diagnostic value of auscultation is a controversial subject. Some believe that bowel sounds have little or no diagnostic value; however, the tinkles and rushes of small bowel obstruction are frequently sought on examinations and clinical rounds. There should always be hepatic dullness to percussion in the right midaxillary line. Resonance in this region is the presence of free air under the diaphragm.

259. The answer is E. *(Isselbacher, 13/e, pp 1509–1512.)* This reaction is a positive Murphy's sign and is found in patients with acute cholecystitis. The anterior abdominal wall is inverted below the right costal margin by the examiner's digital pressure. The liver and gallbladder move inferiorly as the diaphragm contracts on deep inspiration. The inferior movement of the diaphragm causes the inflamed gallbladder to become compressed against the inverted wall. The patient will experience sharp pain and abruptly halt inspiration.

260. The answer is D. *(Sapira, p 376.)* McBurney's point is the point on the abdomen that overlies the anatomic position of the appendix and is the site of maximum tenderness in a patient with acute appendicitis. McBurney himself described it as being "between an inch and a half and two inches from the anterior spinous process of the ileum on a straight line drawn from that process to the umbilicus."

261. The answer is E. *(Seidel, 3/e, p 525.)* This is the clinical picture of a ruptured spleen. Intense pain in the left upper quadrant that radiates to the top of the left shoulder (Kehr's sign) is due to diaphragmatic irritation by blood from the ruptured spleen. The spinal levels supplying most of the sensory fibers of the diaphragm (C3, C4, C5—phrenic nerve) are the same levels as some of the sensory supply to the shoulder; therefore, diaphragmatic irritation will sometimes be perceived as shoulder pain. The blood loss to the abdomen frequently causes signs of shock, including pallor, subnormal temperature, and hypotension. A positive peritoneal lavage is enough to warrant immediate exploratory laparotomy and splenectomy if the ruptured spleen cannot be repaired.

262. The answer is C. *(Sapira, p 374.)* Peritonitis often results in abdominal rigidity (guarding). Findings may range, however, from a persistently stiff, motionless abdomen to stiffness only with palpation to a completely flaccid abdomen. When a patient raises the head from the bed to touch the chin to the chest, the abdominal muscles contract and guarding is induced. This protects the abdominal contents from the palpating hand and may reduce the amount of tenderness elicited by palpation. Rebound tenderness is tested by depressing the abdominal wall and then abruptly withdrawing the examining hand. The abdominal wall passively springs back into place, carrying with it the inflamed peritoneum. The test is positive if the rebound portion of this test causes severe pain. The referred rebound test is conducted in the same fashion but in a location away from the area of tenderness. The patient will experience pain in the area of stated tenderness, rather than the site where the test is performed.

263. The answer is D. *(Seidel, 3/e, pp 524–525. Moore, 3/e, p 210.)* Spider angiomata are commonly found in patients with hepatic disease. Papilledema is associated with intracranial hypertension. Patients with cirrhosis of the liver may develop portal hypertension from obstructed portal blood flow through the liver. In these situations, the portal-systemic anastomoses become clinically important. There are no valves in the portal venous system. As a result, blood is diverted from the portal system to the systemic system by way of the portal-systemic anastomoses. These anastomotic vessels become dilated from increased pressure and are called varicose veins. Tributaries of the left gastric vein anastomose with the esophageal veins, which drain into the azygos vein. When these veins dilate, they are called esophageal varices. The superior rectal vein anastomoses with the middle and inferior rectal veins, which drain into the internal iliac and pudendal veins, respectively. Varicose veins in this region are called hemorrhoids. Paraumbilical veins anastomose with subcutaneous veins of the anterior abdominal wall. Varicose veins in this region lead to a condition called caput medusae. The major clinical manifestations of portal hypertension include hemorrhage from gastroesophageal varices, splenomegaly with hypersplenism, ascites, and acute and chronic hepatic encephalopathy.

264. The answer is C. *(Moore, 3/e, p 405.)* A femoral hernia is a hernia of the femoral canal, which is a continuation of the femoral sheath, through which a small hernia may bulge when intraabdominal pressure is increased. It is much more common in females. The femoral canal is medial to the femoral artery, separated only by the femoral vein, and it therefore presents approximately 2 cm medial to the arterial pulse of the femoral artery.

265. The answer is D. *(Isselbacher, 13/e, p 1423.)* Intestinal ischemia is characterized by the triad of postprandial pain, anorexia (from fear of eating), and weight loss. The pain is typically intermittent and often occurs 30 min after eating and persists from 20 min to 3 h.

266. The answer is A. *(Moore, 3/e, pp 132–149.)* Because of the high prevalence of hernias, a thorough understanding of their diagnosis and differentiation should be attained. A hernia is described as *indirect* if it lies within the inguinal canal. This type of hernia may pass down the canal and present as a mass within the scrotum. The indirect hernia is the most common type of abdominal hernia and is found most often in young men. Since an indirect hernia on one side strongly suggests the possibility of bilateral hernias, the opposite side should be thoroughly examined. A hernia through the posterior wall of the inguinal canal is termed *direct.* The site of the weakness of the wall is Hesselbach's triangle, bounded laterally by the inferior epigastric artery and medially by the lateral border of the rectus abdominis muscle and the inguinal ligament; thus, it lies almost *directly* behind the external inguinal ring. The bulge, therefore, is medial to the site of the bulge of an indirect inguinal hernia. A direct hernia, compared with an indirect hernia, rarely causes pain and is always acquired.

267. The answer is D. *(Seidel, 3/e, pp 488–489.)* Brisk diarrhea or early intestinal obstruction produces increased bowel sounds. Any condition that produces ileus (absence of peristalsis) will have absent bowel sounds. This can occur with peritonitis, mesenteric thrombosis, pneumonia, myxedema, electrolyte abnormalities, spinal cord injuries, and advanced intestinal obstruction.

268. The answer is D. *(Seidel, 3/e, pp 482–521.)* Voluntary rigidity is a sign of resistance to palpation due to reasons such as unrelaxed posture, a chilling external environment, cold hands of the examiner, or fear of painful or ticklish manipulation. Involuntary guarding of abdominal musculature is caused by reflex muscle spasm due to peritoneal irritation. Other signs of peritoneal irritation are rebound tenderness (Blumberg's sign), tenderness to palpation, and tenderness upon vibration (Markel's sign), which can be tested by the heel jar test.

269. The answer is D. *(Sapira, p 371.)* Scaphoid refers to the normal boat-like appearance of the abdomen in thin persons. The costal margins, anterior iliac spines, and pubis represent the sides of the boat while the bottom of the boat is represented by the abdominal wall, which appears sunken in response to the effects of gravity in the supine patient. An obese patient may have an unremarkable abdomen, but it will not be scaphoid. *Scaphoid* denotes an unremarkable abdomen in a patient in whom an abnormal contour would be seen if present, whereas in an obese abdomen, an abnormal contour would be masked by the obesity.

270. The answer is A. *(Bates, 5/e, p 362.)* The span of the normal adult liver is 6 to 12 cm in the midclavicular line and 4 to 8 cm in the midsternal line. The span is generally greater in men than women, and greater in tall people than short people.

271. The answer is B. *(Isselbacher, 13/e, pp 208, 224–225, 1362–1363, 1490–1491.)* Esophageal varices from portal hypertension (due to alcoholic cirrhosis) can rupture and cause frank hematemesis. Mallory-Weiss syndrome is caused by longitudinal tears in the mucosa of the gastroesophageal junction due to prolonged and violent retching or vomiting, frequently associated with alcoholism. If the tear in the gastroesophageal junction is transmural, then it is referred to as *Boerhaave's syndrome.* A bleeding peptic ulcer can also produce hematemesis; however, if the blood has been retained in the stomach, the digestive processes change the hemoglobin to a brown or black pigment, which is commonly referred to as coffee-ground emesis. Esophageal reflux is not associated with hematemesis unless esophageal ulceration has occurred. Esophageal reflux usually presents with a constant, deep, steady, or burning pain in the retrosternal area. These attacks may resemble angina, but are not usually relieved by nitroglycerin.

272. The answer is B. *(Isselbacher, 13/e, pp 526, 1433–1435, 1505–1512.)* When the appendix ruptures, the pain intensifies, vomiting recurs, the temperature rises still higher, and leukocytosis increases. Perforation can form abscesses in the pelvis, which may be localized by demonstrating irritation of the more lateral iliopsoas muscle, or by the medial internal obturator muscle. Rebound tenderness and jar tenderness are tests for peritoneal inflammation and are likely to be positive in a patient with a perforated appendix. A positive Murphy's sign is seen in acute cholecystitis during palpation under the right costal margin and is demonstrated when the patient abruptly arrests inspiration and withdraws in pain when the inflamed gallbladder comes in contact with the examiner's fingers.

273. The answer is D. *(Isselbacher, 13/e, pp 1505–1512.)* Cholelithiasis has an increased incidence in American Indians and in obesity, diabetes, pregnancy, and estrogen use. The ratio of females to males is 4:1. Remember the mnemonic aid of the four *F*'s of increased risk of cholelithiasis: Female, Fat, Forty, and Fertile.

274. The answer is A. *(Isselbacher, 13/e, pp 226–232.)* Jaundice occurs when the serum bilirubin level exceeds 2 to 4 mg/dL. Hyperbilirubinemia may be subclinical in that before it causes visible staining of the skin and sclerae, it can be detected only by blood tests. Bile pigments stain all the tissues of the body; however, this is most pronounced in the face, trunk, and sclerae. Jaundice usually presents as a yellow color, but with prolonged jaundice a greenish color may be noticed owing to oxidation of tissue bilirubin stores to biliverdin. Jaundice from hyperbilirubinemia can be distinguished from high levels of carotenes or quinacrine by the lack of scleral discoloration in the nonbilirubin types of pigmentation.

275. The answer is E. *(Eskelinen, Scand J Gastroenterol 30:349, 1995.)* In multivariate logistic regression analysis, the most significant predictors of acute appendicitis in patients more than 50 years of age were tenderness, rigidity, and pain. The sensitivity of the preoperative clinical decision of acute appendicitis in the aged was 0.87, with a specificity of 0.92. A computer-assisted score improved the sensitivity to 0.92. The authors concluded that acute abdominal pain at the right lower quadrant with tenderness, rigidity, and elevated body temperature is indicative of acute appendicitis in patients more than 50 years of age.

276. The answer is C. *(Isselbacher, 13/e, pp 1363–1378.)* A peptic ulcer (duodenal or gastric) presents with epigastric pain 1 to 4 h postprandially with rhythmicity and periodicity. It is relieved by food, H2 blockers, and alkali (antacid tablets). Its attributes are usually diagnostic. (Recall that attributes of pain are commonly described in the "PQRST" format: P = provoking/palliating factors, Q = quality of the pain, R = region/radiation, S = severity, and T = temporal relations.) A peptic ulcer is commonly provoked by fasting or drinking alcohol or coffee. It is commonly palliated by ingestion of food or alkali. It is usually described as a gnawing, aching, or burning pain. The severity varies from mild to severe. It occurs about 1 to 4 h after meals.

277. The answer is B. *(Isselbacher, 13/e, pp 223–226.)* Hematemesis usually indicates bleeding proximal to the ligament of Treitz. The color of the vomited blood is dependent upon the concentration of blood with respect to hydrochloric acid. If the vomiting occurs shortly after the onset of bleeding, the vomitus will appear red. If the vomiting occurs after the blood has had sufficient exposure to the gastric acid, then the vomitus will have the characteristic coffee-ground appearance. Melena usually denotes bleeding from the upper GI tract; however, lesions in the small intestine and the ascending colon may rarely produce melena provided the GI transit time is sufficiently prolonged. Approximately 60 mL of blood is required to produce a single black stool. Hematochezia, the passage of red blood per rectum, is generally from bleeding at a site distal to the ligament of Treitz; however, if an upper GI hemorrhage is rapid enough, it may also result in hematochezia. A diverticular hemorrhage usually presents as a painless passage of a maroon-colored stool.

278. The answer is D. *(Isselbacher, 13/e, pp 1437–1504, 2336.)* Physical examination of patients with chronic liver failure commonly demonstrates palmar erythema, spider angiomata, jaundice, Dupuytren's contractures, peripheral neuritis, and enlargement of the parotid and lacrimal glands. There is also clinical evidence of hypogonadism and overt feminization with gynecomastia and development of a female escutcheon and body habitus in males with cirrhosis.

279. The answer is C. *(Sapira, pp 382–383.)* A palpable liver is not necessarily enlarged. Using palpability as a sign of enlargement has a 54 percent false positive rate. Determining the size of the liver requires percussion, the scratch test, or auscultatory percussion. The liver may be easily palpated in patients with a depressed diaphragm secondary to hyperinflation of emphysematous lungs. A stony, hard liver is usually due to tumor, and when nodules are found by palpation they are usually due to cancer rather than nodular cirrhosis. A moderately hard liver with a sharp edge is usually cirrhotic. In the course of alcohol-induced cirrhosis, the liver is usually enlarged and firm in the early stages, but later may be of normal size or even small. Expansive systolic pulsations are frequently discussed as a sign of tricuspid insufficiency or aortic insufficiency; however, some authors feel that most true hepatic expansile pulsations (as distinct from false positives due to misinterpretations of aortic pulse transmission) are actually presystolic hepatic venous pulsations.

280. The answer is A. *(Harvey, 22/e, p 792.)* The hallmarks of intestinal obstruction are abdominal pain, distention, vomiting, and obstipation. Symptoms vary in intensity depending on the level of obstruction. An obstruction high in the small intestine commonly produces copious vomiting, while an obstruction in the colon may present with distention as the major symptom. On physical examination, the abdomen is usually distended and bowel sounds are typically high-pitched and occur in rushes. In late stages of obstruction, bowel sounds may be diminished or absent. Ascites is not commonly found in obstruction; it is usually associated with abnormal liver function or low plasma oncotic pressure

281. The answer is A. *(Sapira, pp 384–386.)* The spleen, as well as the liver and gallbladder, should descend upon inspiration. If a spleen is found on palpation to be hard, the splenomegaly is fibrotic and thus chronic in nature, as in 44 percent of patients with Laennec's cirrhosis. If the spleen is merely tense (like an uncooked hot dog), then the splenomegaly is acute. When splenomegaly is accompanied by jaundice, this indicates either hepatic disease with portal hypertension or a hemolytic anemia. Massive splenomegaly is seen in a number of conditions, including chronic granulocytic leukemia, polycythemia vera, Hodgkin's disease, myeloid metaplasia, and malaria. Patients with sickle cell disease commonly have small spleens caused by autosplenectomy secondary to repeated infarcts. Patients with functional asplenia are prone to overwhelming infection by encapsulated bacteria and should be appropriately vaccinated.

282. The answer is C. *(Burnside, 17/e, p 232.)* Vascular sounds in the abdomen indicate areas of turbulent flow, which can be found in dilated, constricted, or tortuous vessels. Where the bruit is heard best can be a good indicator of the source of the bruit; however, definitive localization of the bruit is dependent upon arteriography. Bruits of the aorta are heard best in the right hypochondrium. Bruits of the splenic artery are heard best in the left hypochondrium. Renal artery bruits are heard best in the umbilical region, in the flanks, and occasionally in the costovertebral angles. In patients with hypertension, these bruits may indicate renal artery stenosis. Finally, vascular bruits can be distinguished from transmitted heart murmurs by simultaneously palpating the cardiac apex while listening to the bruit. The transmitted murmur will be synchronous with the impulse, whereas a local bruit occurs somewhat later.

283. The answer is E. *(Isselbacher, 13/e, pp 1336–1338.)* Renal cell carcinoma has been called the "internist's tumor" because of its systemic rather than its urologic manifestations. The triad of gross hematuria, flank pain, and a palpable abdominal mass, although considered classic evidence for the clinical diagnosis, is encountered in less than 10 percent of cases. The most common presenting abnormality is hematuria, which is found in 60 percent of the cases. Systemic symptoms of fatigability, weight loss, and cachexia occur in about 50 percent of patients. Intermittent fever unassociated with infection occurs occasionally and may be the only presenting symptom. Anemia is present in approximately 50 percent of the cases. Renal cell carcinomas may also produce hormones that in turn may produce hypercalcemia, galactorrhea, hypertension, feminization, masculinization, or Cushing's syndrome.

284. The answer is A. *(Isselbacher, 13/e, pp 224–226, 1424–1433.)* Lesions of the right colon commonly ulcerate, which leads to chronic, insidious blood loss without a change in the appearance of the stools. Consequently, patients with tumors of the ascending colon often present with symptoms such as fatigue and palpitations and are found to have a hypochromic, microcytic anemia indicative of iron deficiency. Stool is relatively liquid as it passes through the right colon; however, it becomes more concentrated as it progresses into the transverse and descending colon. Thus, tumors arising in the left colon tend to impede the passage of stool and may present with a picture of obstruction and even perforation. Radiographs of the abdomen often reveal the characteristic annular constricting lesions ("apple-core," or "napkin ring"). Neoplasms of the rectosigmoid often are associated with hematochezia, tenesmus, and narrowing in the caliber of the stool; nonetheless, anemia is an infrequent finding.

285. The answer is E. *(Isselbacher, 13/e, pp 62, 78, 1122, 1132–1133.)* Atherosclerosis is the predominant cause of abdominal aortic aneurysms. Frequently these aneurysms are found while one examines a patient who presents with low back pain. On physical examination an expansile, pulsating mass can be palpated between the umbilicus and xiphoid process. Since the aorta is anchored, the mass cannot be moved cephalad or caudad. A bruit can only be detected in about 10 percent of cases. A sonogram of the abdomen or an abdominal CT scan would be the next diagnostic step.

286–289. The answers are 286-B, 287-C, 288-D, 289-A. *(Bates, 5/e, p 256.)* Dullness to percussion is heard over fluid or solid tissue. Resonance is heard over normal lung. If dullness replaces the resonance of normal lung, disease should be suspected (e.g., lobar pneumonia, pleural effusion, hemothorax, empyema, fibrosis, or tumor). Hyperresonance is heard over the hyperinflated lungs of emphysema or asthma. Unilateral hyperresonance would suggest a large pneumothorax. Tympany is heard over hollow organs, such as a gas-filled stomach or bowel.

290–293. The answers are 290-B, 291-C, 292-D, 293-A. *(Seidel, 3/e, pp 504–507, 725–726.)* The words that patients use to characterize their pain may be very valuable in making a preliminary diagnosis. Different pathologic processes commonly elicit different pain characteristics. A "burning" pain is commonly associated with lesions secondary to acidic erosion, such as peptic ulcers or esophageal reflux. A history of relief with eating or use of antacids is also common. "Cramping" is a word used often in cases of gastric or intestinal disease, especially disease that involves obstruction of hollow viscera. Acute pancreatitis commonly presents with the history of a "knifelike," mid-epigastric pain that may radiate through to the back. A gradual onset of pain is usually suggestive of an infectious or neoplastic process.

294–298. The answers are 294-C, 295-B, 296-E, 297-A, 298-D. *(Bates, 5/e, p 96.)* The specific location of abdominal pain is very useful in establishing the probable underlying pathology. Early appendicitis commonly begins as a poorly localized periumbilical pain prior to becoming localized to the right lower quadrant.

Meckel's diverticulitis usually presents with pain of the right lower quadrant. (Remember the rule of 2's with Meckel's diverticulae: Present in 2 percent of the population, 2 feet proximal to the cecum, and 2 inches long.) Sigmoid diverticulitis, owing to its anatomic position, presents most commonly with pain of the left lower quadrant.

A duodenal ulcer should be included in the differential diagnosis in patients with pain of the right upper quadrant, although cholecystitis and hepatitis should be suspected first.

Pain of the left upper quadrant is a common finding in patients with a ruptured spleen; however, there may also be generalized abdominal pain with guarding and rebound secondary to peritoneal irritation from the blood released into the abdomen. Diaphragmatic irritation may produce pain referred to the left shoulder (Kehr's sign).

299–302. The answers are 299-B, 300-C, 301-A, 302-E. *(Sapira, pp 371–389.)* The appearance of the undisturbed patient can provide valuable information to the examining physician. Although not always correct, a good rule of thumb is that patients with peritonitis are motionless whereas those with obstruction are restless. Patients with peritonitis are made more uncomfortable during movement that irritates the inflamed peritoneum. With a perinephric abscess, patients may find relief with bending toward the affected side, whereas bending away from the affected side aggravates the pain. Caput medusae is a prominent venous pattern seen in some patients with portal hypertension. The veins radiate out from the umbilicus. In patients with inferior vena caval obstruction, the veins do not radiate from the umbilicus but rather from the inferior to superior.

303–306. The answers are 303-B, 304-D, 305-C, 306-A. *(Isselbacher, 13/e, pp 1422, 1513, 1533. Sapira, p 386.)* Courvoisier's law states that a palpable, nontender gallbladder in a jaundiced patient suggests neoplastic destruction of the common duct, most often due to pancreatic cancer. This finding is present in about half the cases. The underlying theory is that the severely scarred gallbladder of chronic cholecystitis cannot expand, but the one acutely obstructed by neoplasm can.

Dance's sign is pathognomonic for intussusception. It is the presence of a palpable oblong mass in the right or upper mid abdomen and an absence of bowel sounds in the right lower quadrant.

The hallmark of mesenteric artery obstruction is pain out of proportion to the physical findings. The onset is sudden with agonizing pain between the xiphoid and umbilicus that is often not relieved by narcotics. In 50 percent of the cases there is a positive history of intestinal ischemia. Hypothermia and hypotension result, as well as a profound metabolic acidosis. Prognosis is poor.

Ascending cholangitis is defined by Charcot's triad, which is abdominal pain, fever and chills, and jaundice. It is a bacterial infection of the biliary ducts in the setting of biliary obstruction.

307–310. The answers are 307-B, 308-D, 309-A, 310-C. *(Isselbacher, 13/e, pp 211, 1355–1360, 1366, 1378–1382.)* Heartburn is the characteristic symptom of reflux esophagitis, which may mimic the pain of angina. Reflux esophagitis commonly demonstrates a diurnal pattern in which pain often occurs nocturnally and with recumbency, especially after a large meal. Increased gastric pressure overcomes the lower esophageal sphincter and reflux occurs.

Gastric outlet obstruction commonly presents as late postprandial pain. It usually occurs several hours after eating, which reflects the failure of the stomach to empty adequately.

Acute gastritis usually demonstrates early postprandial pain, which is due to irritation of the inflamed mucosa by the food and subsequent secretion of acid.

Duodenal ulcers characteristically present with the relief of pain following ingestion of food or antacids. This is presumably due to the neutralization of the acidic environment.

311–316. The answers are 311-A, 312-B, 313-D, 314-B, 315-A, 316-B. *(Isselbacher, 13/e, pp 603, 1403–1417.)* The major symptoms of ulcerative colitis are bloody diarrhea and abdominal pain, often with fever and weight loss in more severe cases. The major clinical features of Crohn's disease are fever, abdominal pain, diarrhea often without blood, and generalized fatigability. Rectal bleeding is distinctly less common in Crohn's disease than in ulcerative colitis and reflects (1) the sparing of the rectum in many patients and (2) the transmural nature of Crohn's disease, which has only irregular mucosal involvement. In Crohn's disease there may be severe complications such as fistulas, fissures, and perirectal abscesses. Physical examination of patients with Crohn's disease often reveals tenderness of the right lower quadrant with an associated fullness or mass that reflects adherent loops of bowel. There are increasing reports of small bowel and colonic malignancy in the setting of long-standing Crohn's disease. Although the risk of developing a malignancy is statistically increased, this complication is uncommon when compared with the frequency of malignancy in ulcerative colitis. Pseudomembranous colitis (antibiotic-associated colitis) is caused by a necrolytic toxin elaborated by *Clostridium difficile*, which proliferates in the bowel secondary to a disturbance of the normal bowel flora associated with the use of antibiotics.

Musculoskeletal System

DIRECTIONS: Each item below contains a question or incomplete statement followed by suggested responses. Select the **one best** response to each question.

317. An obese 60-year-old woman presents with progressive pain and swelling of the right knee of 12 months' duration. Her symptoms are worse after activity and late in the day. She has little pain or stiffness in the mornings. No other joints are involved and she is otherwise in good health. Your working diagnosis is

(A) Reiter's syndrome
(B) gout
(C) rheumatoid arthritis
(D) osteoarthritis
(E) psoriatic arthritis

318. Which of the following findings is typical in a patient with congenital radioulnar synostosis?

(A) Unsteady gait
(B) Fixed pronation of forearm
(C) Poor wrist mobility
(D) Hypermobility of the elbow
(E) Tenderness over the distal metacarpal bones

319. A 16-year-old wrestler sustains an elbow injury when he is thrown to the matt on his outstretched left arm. His elbow seemed to be dislocated, then spontaneously reduced with the help of his coach. Since this event, the patient has noted three additional episodes of instability that reduces with minimal effort by the patient or parent. On examination the elbow is stable to varus and valgus stress. Which test or maneuver will likely diagnose this condition?

(A) Valgus stress radiograph
(B) Varus stress radiograph
(C) Tinel's sign
(D) Finkelstein's test
(E) Posterolateral rotatory instability test

320. A 1-year-old boy is brought to the clinic with a tentative diagnosis of congenital muscular torticollis. All the following would be consistent with this diagnosis EXCEPT

(A)   decreased range of motion of the cervical spine
(B)   tilt of the head to the side of the muscle involved
(C)   rotation of the head so that the chin points to the side of the involved muscle
(D)   asymmetry of the skull and facial bones
(E)   a history of a mass in the sternocleidomastoid muscle

321. The initial screening test for scoliosis would include which of the following?

(A)   Growth charts
(B)   Lateral x-ray
(C)   Forward bending test
(D)   Gaenslen's test
(E)   None of the above

322. Which of the following is true of a patient who arises by using the arms to push off from the legs?

(A)   The patient likely has a brainstem injury
(B)   The patient likely has a cerebellar injury
(C)   The patient is demonstrating a positive Tinel's sign
(D)   This is a positive sign for a congenital defect
(E)   This response is pathognomonic for Duchenne's muscular dystrophy

323. A young man is brought to your office with a fracture of the humerus in its distal third. He is unable to extend his wrist. What structure is most likely damaged?

(A)   Brachial vessel
(B)   Radial nerve
(C)   Median nerve
(D)   Ulnar nerve
(E)   Axillary nerve

324. All the following would be consistent with Legg-Calvé-Perthes disease EXCEPT

(A)   insidious onset of groin pain
(B)   onset at 16 years of age
(C)   worsening of pain with activity
(D)   short stature for age
(E)   limited hip abduction and internal rotation

325. Pain reproduced by extending the wrist against resistance with the elbow extended is most suggestive of

(A)   olecranon bursitis
(B)   tennis elbow
(C)   golfer's elbow
(D)   osteoarthritis
(E)   biceps tendinitis

326. Chronic stenosing tenosynovitis (DeQuervain's disease) is effectively diagnosed via

(A)   Finkelstein's test
(B)   Radiography
(C)   Tinel's sign
(D)   Mill's maneuver
(E)   none of the above

327. Intervertebral disk protrusion at the level of L4-L5 would be likely to cause all the following EXCEPT

(A) pain of the hip and lateral thigh
(B) decreased ankle jerk
(C) weakness of the extensor hallucis longus
(D) paresthesias of the lateral calf
(E) weakness of dorsiflexion of the foot

328. A 25-year-old man presents with morning back pain, stiffness and tenderness over the sacroiliac joints, and diminished chest expansion. The most likely diagnosis is

(A) rheumatoid arthritis
(B) ankylosing spondylitis
(C) Sjögren's syndrome
(D) systemic lupus erythematosus

329. *Knock knee* describes which of the following deviations?

(A) Genu varum
(B) Genu valgum
(C) Genu recurvatum
(D) Genu impressum
(E) None of the above

330. A patient with rheumatoid arthritis presents with a painful midline swelling of the popliteal fossa that is visible only when the knee is extended. This is most likely

(A) a Baker's cyst
(B) a cyst of the lateral meniscus
(C) a cyst of the medial meniscus
(D) anserine bursitis
(E) infrapatellar bursitis

331. A young adult male presents with arthritis, skin lesions, and acute tenosynovitis. Which of the following is the most likely diagnosis?

(A) Disseminated gonococcal infection
(B) DeQuervain's stenosing tenosynovitis
(C) Acute pseudogout
(D) Osteoarthritis
(E) Reiter's syndrome

332. Hypovolemic shock and life-threatening blood loss would be most likely to occur with fracture of the

(A) femur
(B) spine
(C) pelvis
(D) tibia
(E) radius

333. All the following peripheral nerves and function tests are correctly paired EXCEPT

(A) femoral nerve (L2-L4), knee extension
(B) axillary nerve (C5, C6), shoulder abduction
(C) radial nerve (C6-C8), thumb extension
(D) musculocutaneous nerve (C5, C6), elbow extension

334. Muscle atrophy is associated with

(A) motor nerve loss
(B) hypothyroidism
(C) overuse
(D) congenital myotonia
(E) none of the above

335. Sagging of the unsupported hemipelvis is characteristic of all the following EXCEPT

(A) a positive Trendelenburg's sign
(B) paralysis of the gluteal muscle
(C) gluteal muscle weakness
(D) fibrous ankylosis of the hip

336. Ballottement of the patella causes a palpable tap or clicking in all the following EXCEPT

(A) joint effusion
(B) hemarthrosis
(C) hydrarthrosis
(D) infrapatellar bursitis
(E) suppurative arthritis

337. A football player is tackled from the side with his foot planted, which causes a forced valgus bending of the knee. On examination, you elicit a forward movement of the tibia of 2 cm on the anterior drawer test. All the following findings would be consistent with this history and examination EXCEPT

(A) rupture of the tibial (medial) collateral ligament
(B) rupture of the medial meniscus
(C) rupture of the anterior cruciate ligament
(D) rupture of the posterior cruciate ligament
(E) hemarthrosis

338. Sprengel's deformity can be characterized by which of the following statements?

(A) The neck on the affected side appears full
(B) It involves pain of the elbow and wrist
(C) Limited abduction of the hip is the principal sign
(D) It generally affects elderly patients
(E) None of the above

339. A 60-year-old man involved in an automobile accident suffered multiple long-bone fractures and injury to the pelvis. Two days following his admission, he was febrile with sinus tachycardia, axillary and conjunctival petechiae, and a P_{O_2} of 64 mmHg. Your working diagnosis is

(A) gram-negative sepsis with ARDS
(B) fat embolism syndrome
(C) lower lobe pneumonia
(D) acute exacerbation of COPD
(E) anemia

340. Which of the following statements is true of glenohumeral dislocations?

(A) Most are posterior dislocations
(B) The normal curvature of the shoulder is seldom affected
(C) They usually result from forced abduction and external rotation
(D) The head of the humerus lies superior to the coracoid process
(E) The acromion is less prominent

341. A woman presents with a pathologic process that involves the hip joint. When asked to identify the site of pain, she would most likely point to the

(A) groin
(B) knee
(C) posterior aspect of the greater trochanter
(D) buttock
(E) calf

342. Which of the following statements is true of the crossed straight-leg raising test?

(A) Straight-leg raising of the non-painful leg causes ipsilateral pain
(B) Straight-leg raising of the non-painful leg causes worsened pain on the painful side
(C) Straight-leg raising of the painful leg causes pain on the nonpainful side
(D) Straight-leg raising of the painful leg causes pain on both sides
(E) None of the above

DIRECTIONS: Each group of questions below consists of lettered options followed by numbered items. For each numbered item, select the appropriate lettered option(s). Each lettered option may be used once, more than once, or not at all. **Choose exactly the number of options indicated following each item.**

Items 343–347

Match the disorders below with the appropriate signs.

(A) Short fingers of almost equal length
(B) Ulnar deviation
(C) Wristdrop
(D) Clawhand
(E) Thenar atrophy

343. Paralyzed interosseus and lumbrical muscles due to an ulnar nerve injury **(SELECT 1 SIGN)**

344. Achondroplasia **(SELECT 1 SIGN)**

345. Rheumatoid arthritis **(SELECT 1 SIGN)**

346. Radial nerve palsy **(SELECT 1 SIGN)**

347. Lesions of the median nerve **(SELECT 1 SIGN)**

Items 348–352

Match each description with the appropriate condition.

(A) Dupuytren's contracture
(B) Mallet finger
(C) Ganglion
(D) Carpal tunnel syndrome
(E) Boxer's fracture

348. A fibrotic process of the palmar fascia **(SELECT 1 CONDITION)**

349. A painless, firm cystic mass arising from the wrist joint **(SELECT 1 CONDITION)**

350. Flexion deformity of the distal interphalangeal joint **(SELECT 1 CONDITION)**

351. A positive Tinel's sign **(SELECT 1 CONDITION)**

352. Flattening or loss of the fifth knuckle prominence **(SELECT 1 CONDITION)**

Items 353–357

Match the signs and symptoms below with the correct condition.

(A) Reiter's syndrome
(B) Bicipital tendinitis
(C) Anterior shoulder dislocation
(D) Rotator cuff tendinitis
(E) Paralysis of the long thoracic nerve

353. Pain on resisted supination (Yergason's sign) **(SELECT 1 CONDITION)**

354. Severe pain on abduction **(SELECT 1 CONDITION)**

355. Circinate balanitis **(SELECT 1 CONDITION)**

356. Winged scapula **(SELECT 1 CONDITION)**

357. Flattening of the shoulder profile and inability to adduct the arm sufficiently to touch the opposite shoulder **(SELECT 1 CONDITION)**

Items 358–362

Match the following.

(A) Bunions
(B) Hammer toe
(C) Swan-neck deformity
(D) Gout
(E) March fracture

358. Hallux valgus **(SELECT 1 CONDITION)**

359. Rheumatoid arthritis of the hand **(SELECT 1 CONDITION)**

360. Permanent flexion of the proximal interphalangeal joint **(SELECT 1 CONDITION)**

361. Excessive walking **(SELECT 1 CONDITION)**

362. Painful swelling of the metatarsophalangeal joint of the great toe **(SELECT 1 CONDITION)**

Items 363–367

Match the following.

(A) Juvenile rheumatoid arthritis
(B) Rickets
(C) Osgood-Schlatter disease
(D) Torn meniscus
(E) Muscular dystrophy

363. Progressive weakness **(SELECT 1 CONDITION)**

364. Pain in the region of the tibial tuberosity **(SELECT 1 CONDITION)**

365. Pericarditis **(SELECT 1 CONDITION)**

366. Rachitic rosary (beads) **(SELECT 1 CONDITION)**

367. Catching or locking sensation **(SELECT 1 CONDITION)**

Items 368–372

Match each description below with the appropriate test.

(A) Ortolani's test
(B) Barlow's test
(C) Telescoping test
(D) Allis' test
(E) Ober's test

368. Used to evaluate iliotibial band tension **(SELECT 1 TEST)**

369. Conducted by exerting an anteriorly directed force on the proximal femur **(SELECT 1 TEST)**

370. Positive in a patient with an unstable but well-located hip joint **(SELECT 1 TEST)**

371. Performed by applying anterior and posterior longitudinal forces on the femur **(SELECT 1 TEST)**

372. Positive in a patient with a discrepancy of leg length **(SELECT 1 TEST)**

Items 373–374

Match each patient with the likely diagnoses.

(A) Carpal tunnel syndrome
(B) Posterior interosseus nerve palsy
(C) Trigger finger
(D) Rupture of extensor pollicis longus tendon
(E) Rupture of extensor digitorum tendon to small finger
(F) Rupture of extensor digiti minimi tendon
(G) Subluxation of extensor tendon between metacarpal heads

373. A 60-year-old woman presents with rheumatoid arthritis. She awakes several times each night with numbness and tingling in her left hand and thumb and index fingers. Her right ring finger locks in the flexed position. With assistance from her left hand, the right ring finger extends with a "pop," or snapping action. **(SELECT TWO DIAGNOSES)**

374. The patient in the question above returns 6 months later and has difficulty extending her fingers. She cannot obtain but can maintain metacarpophalangeal (MCP) extension of the left index finger. On the right she can actively extend all digits. When the MCP joints of the index, long, and ring fingers are held in flexion, she is unable to extend the small finger. **(SELECT TWO DIAGNOSES)**

DIRECTIONS: Each group of questions below consists of four lettered options followed by a set of numbered items. For each numbered item select

A	if the item is associated with	(A) only
B	if the item is associated with	(B) only
C	if the item is associated with	**both** (A) and (B)
D	if the item is associated with	**neither** (A) nor (B)

Each lettered option may be used **once, more than once, or not at all.**

Items 375–377

(A) Afflictions of the hip joint
(B) Irritation of the sciatic nerve
(C) Both
(D) Neither

375. Pain produced on straight-leg raising test at 40° of elevation with knee extended

376. Pain produced on straight-leg raising test at 40° of elevation, which is relieved by flexing the knee joint

377. Pain produced on the straight-leg raising test, which is relieved by dorsiflexion of the foot

Items 378–379

(A) Test of integrity of the flexor digitorum superficialis tendons
(B) Test of integrity of the flexor digitorum profundus tendons
(C) Both
(D) Neither

378. The hand is placed on the examination table with the palm facing up and the examiner holds the metacarpophalangeal joint and proximal interphalangeal joint in full extension while the patient flexes the distal interphalangeal joint

379. The hand is placed on the examination table with the palm facing up and the examiner holds the uninvolved fingers in full extension while the patient flexes the finger to be tested

Musculoskeletal System

Answers

317. The answer is D. *(Gartland, 4/e, p 122. Isselbacher, 13/e, p 1695.)* Osteoarthritis most often affects large weight-bearing joints and is associated with obesity or other forms of mechanical stress. It is more common in women and onset is usually after the age of 50. Pain often occurs on exertion and is relieved by rest, after which the involved joint may become stiff. Distal interphalangeal joints may be involved with production of Heberden's nodes. Rheumatoid arthritis is inflammatory in nature and is a systemic disease also more common in women, but it has an onset usually before the age of 40. Joint involvement is generally symmetric and often involves proximal interphalangeal and metacarpophalangeal joints. Morning stiffness lasting longer than 30 min is characteristic of rheumatoid arthritis. Ninety-five percent of gouty arthritis occurs in men and often involves the great toe. Aspiration of urate crystals from the joint space or relief following colchicine therapy is diagnostic. Reiter's syndrome is characterized by the triad of arthritis, urethritis, and conjunctivitis. Asymmetric oligoarthritis that involves the knees, ankles, shoulders, or digits of the hands or feet occurs in 50 percent of patients with psoriasis. Nail pitting is generally present in psoriasis.

318. The answer is B. *(Simmons, J Hand Surg 8:829–838, 1983.)* Congenital radioulnar synostosis is a rare malformation of the upper limb in which the proximal aspects of the radius and ulna are fused. The forearm is typically fixed in a pronated position. The children have hypermobility of the wrist, presumably secondary to continued stress due to absence of forearm rotation. Patients may compensate by rotation at the shoulder to obtain enough supination for activities such as accepting coins and feeding themselves. The amount of disability is determined by the amount of fixed forearm pronation. Sixty percent of patients have bilateral involvement. Treatment is surgical derotation of the forearm to a more functional position.

319. The answer is E. *(O'Driscoll, Clin Orthop 280:186–197, 1992.)* The history and finding of this patient are typical of a patient with posterolateral rotatory instability of the elbow. Posterolateral rotatory subluxation is the first stage of the clinical spectrum of acute and recurrent elbow instability (excluding pure valgus and radioulnar mechanisms). Posterolateral rotatory instability of the elbow results from disruption of the lateral ulnar collateral ligament (ulnar part of radial collateral ligament). This allows transient rotatory subluxation of the radiohumeral joint. The mechanism of injury is an axial load, valgus stress, and forearm supination. The posterolateral rotatory instability test involves supination of the forearm and application of a valgus stress and axial compression force across the elbow while it is flexed from a position of full extension. The elbow is reduced in full extension and is subluxated as it is flexed in order to obtain a positive test result. Flexion of more than about 40° produces a palpable and visible reduction of the radial head. Without anesthesia, apprehension is elicited from the patient.

320. The answer is C. *(Morrissy, 4/e, pp 751–754.)* In congenital muscular torticollis (congenital wryneck), rotation of the head is away from the affected side. The condition is due to contracture of the sternocleidomastoid muscle. The head is tilted toward the involved side and the head is rotated so that the chin points to the contralateral side. A mass or tumor may be found (usually within the first 4 months of life) attached to or located within the body of the sternocleidomastoid muscle. Asymmetry of the face and skull may also be present. A history of a difficult or breech delivery may be found; however, many of these cases follow normal, atraumatic deliveries. Although the wryneck posture is most commonly caused by congenital muscular torticollis, other conditions lead to this posture, notably abnormalities of the cervical spine at C1-C2. Approximately 20 percent of children with congenital muscular torticollis have an associated congenital dysplasia of the hip. Therefore, a thorough and complete examination and evaluation are indicated for infants presenting with wryneck deformity.

321. The answer is C. *(Sapira, p 424.)* Vertebral rotation that accompanies structural scoliosis causes a paraspinous prominence (rib hump) when the patient bends forward in full flexion. Radiographic evaluation is used to determine the degree of scoliosis. The Gaenslen's test is performed by hyperextending the hip: pain occurs in lumbosacral disease and sacroiliitis.

322. The answer is D. *(Morrissy, 4/e, pp 540–555.)* Gowers' sign is a series of maneuvers performed by a patient with pelvic and trunk weakness. The patient uses the upper extremities to push off from the lower extremities to compensate for weakness of the proximal muscles of the lower extremity. This sign may be positive in congenital myopathies, spinal muscular atrophy, Duchenne's muscular dystrophy, or any other condition that causes weakness of the pelvic and trunk muscles.

323. The answer is B. *(Crenshaw, 8/e, pp 2227, 2254, 3109, 3118.)* The radial nerve lies next to the shaft of the humerus in the spiral groove. It may be injured as a result of humeral fractures, particularly those involving the distal third of the humerus. The radial nerve supplies the extensor muscles of the wrist and its damage results in wristdrop, a condition in which the patient is unable to extend the wrist.

324. The answer is B. *(Thompson, Orthop Clin North Am 18:617–635.)* Legg-Calvé-Perthes is an uncommon disease generally affecting boys more than girls between the ages of 2 and 12, with a mean of 7 years. The hallmark is avascular necrosis of the capital femoral epiphysis, which has the potential to regenerate with new bone. The bone age of affected children is typically delayed by 1 to 3 years. Consequently, they are shorter than normal children of the same age. Children with Legg-Calvé-Perthes disease present with a limp, pain of the anterior thigh or knee, and limited hip motion, especially abduction and internal rotation.

325. The answer is B. *(Crenshaw, 8/e, pp 1756–1763, 1953. Gartland, 4/e, p 145.)* Tennis elbow is most commonly characterized by tenderness of the common extensor muscles at their origin, the lateral epicondyle of the humerus. Having the patient extend the wrist against resistance causes pain. Passive flexion of the fingers and wrist causes tension of the extensor muscles and pain. Golfer's elbow is a similar disorder of the common flexor muscle group at its origin, the medial epicondyle of the humerus. Olecranon bursitis is an inflammation of the bursa over the olecranon process. Swelling of this bursa may be caused by chronic or acute trauma or may be secondary to gout, rheumatoid arthritis, or infection. Clinically there is swelling or pain to palpation or both. Repetitive minor trauma caused by leaning on the elbow may result in chronic enlargement, also known as bartender's elbow.

326. The answer is A. *(Isselbacher, 13/e, p 1298.)* The first dorsal compartment of the wrist contains the abductor pollicis longus and extensor pollicis brevis tendons. Inflammation of these tendon sheaths may occur with repetitive use, resulting in marked pain and tenderness in the region. Finkelstein's test for tenosynovitis is performed by having the patient make a fist over the flexed thumb. The examiner pushes the base of the flexed thumb forcefully in an ulnar direction, resulting in ulnar deviation of the wrist. When pain is elicited in the region of the radial styloid process as compared with the asymptomatic side, the test is positive.

327. The answer is B. *(Crenshaw, 8/e, pp 3717–3720, 3753–3756.)* The most common levels of disk herniation are L4-L5 and L5-S1, followed by L3-L4. The herniated disk usually affects the nerve root below the lesion. For example, an L4-L5 disk protrusion would compress the fifth lumbar nerve root. Weakness of the quadriceps and decreased knee jerk reflex generally occur with protrusion of the L3-L4 disk but may also occur at the L4-L5 level. Protrusion of the L4-L5 disk produces pain over the sacroiliac joint, hip, lateral thigh, and leg. Numbness may occur on the anterior lateral leg and the web space between the great and second toe. Weakness may be noted on dorsiflexion of the great toe and foot. Diminished ankle jerk is generally seen with protrusion at the L5-S1 level.

328. The answer is B. *(Isselbacher, 13/e, pp 1664–1667.)* Ankylosing spondylitis is a chronic and progressive inflammatory disease that most commonly affects spinal, sacroiliac, and hip joints. Men in the third decade of life are most frequently affected. There is a strong association with HLA-B27. Patients in advanced stages present with a characteristic bent-over posture. A positive Schober test indicates diminished anterior flexion of the lumbar spine. Involvement of the costovertebral joints limits chest expansion.

329. The answer is B. *(Gartland, 4/e, pp 381–382.)* Genu valgum involves the lateral deviation of the leg from the midline so that the medial malleoli are separated when the knees are placed together. In genu varum (bowleg) the medial femoral condyles are widely separated when the feet are placed together in the extended position. In genu recurvatum the knee hyperextends. In genu impressum there is flattening and bending of the knee to one side with displacement of the patella.

330. The answer is A. *(Tintinalli, 4/e, p 1317.)* A Baker's cyst occurs in the midline of the popliteal fossa. It is often a complication of rheumatoid arthritis. The cyst represents a diverticulum of the synovial sac that protrudes through the joint capsule of the knee.

331. The answer is A. *(Isselbacher, 13/e, p 556.)* Gonococcal infection is the leading cause of bacterial arthritis in young adults and the most common form of infectious arthritis seen in urban medical centers. In fact, arthritis may be the only presenting complaint. An early tenosynovitis-dermatitis syndrome is typically followed by septic arthritis. The knee, shoulder, wrist and interphalangeal joints of the hand are most commonly affected. The history and examination should focus on the urogenital tract, pharynx, and rectum in search of a primary focus.

332. The answer is C. *(Tintinalli, 4/e, p 1250.)* The greatest amount of blood loss generally occurs in fractures of the pelvis, followed by those of the femur and spine. Patients with pelvic fractures should be evaluated for hypovolemic shock. Common manifestations include tachycardia, hypotension, oliguria, a clouded sensorium, and cool extremities.

333. The answer is D. *(Pansky, 6/e, pp 248–260.)* A sound knowledge of the function of the peripheral nervous system is helpful in localizing disease. The musculocutaneous nerve (C5-C7) supplies the anterior compartment of the arm and is responsible for flexion of the elbow. The radial nerve (C5-C8) innervates the muscles that extend the elbow, wrist, and fingers.

334. The answer is A. *(Isselbacher, 13/e, p 117.)* Disuse and loss of innervation are common causes of muscle atrophy. Atrophy of the thenar eminence is common in late carpal tunnel syndrome. Hypothyroidism and congenital myotonia are associated with muscle hypertrophy.

335. The answer is D. *(Pansky, 6/e, p 578 .)* A positive Trendelenburg's sign is sagging of the unsupported hemipelvis when the patient is supporting all of his or her weight on one leg. It is seen in gluteal nerve damage or other causes of gluteal muscle weakness. Fibrous ankylosis of the hip is a painful immobility of the hip. A Trendelenburg's sign is not present in fibrous ankylosis of the hip.

336. The answer is D. *(Munro, 9/e, pp 308–309.)* A palpable tap or click on ballottement occurs with fluid in the knee joint. It may be excess synovial fluid (effusion, hydrarthrosis), blood (hemarthrosis), or pus (suppurative arthritis). The patella is separated from the femur by fluid under pressure and therefore clicks when it strikes the femur during the ballottement test. The click or tap may be very subtle; however, the examiner can generally appreciate an intervening space between the patella and the femur. Small effusions will often result in a negative patellar tap test and may be best detected by inspection. When compared with the normal side, an increased fullness, which results in partial obliteration of the hollow along the medial and lateral sides of the patella, may be noted. With greater effusion into the knee, the suprapatellar pouch becomes distended. The fluid displacement test is helpful in detecting a small effusion. Gentle stroking of one side of the joint capsule results in distention of the other side when an effusion is present. The examiner should be careful not to push the patella over, which may result in an incorrect interpretation and a false positive test. A careful history is helpful in distinguishing the type of fluid present. A history of trauma suggests hemarthrosis if the fluid appears hours after trauma or an effusion due to acute traumatic synovitis if the fluid accumulates more slowly (days).

337. The answer is D. *(Crenshaw, 8/e, p 2328. Torg, Am J Sports Med 4:84–93, 1976.)* Forced valgus bending of the knee may rupture the medial collateral ligament. The medial collateral ligament is firmly attached to the medial meniscus, which is often torn as a result. Rupture of the anterior cruciate ligament is associated with violent knee injuries and results in extreme pain followed by hemarthrosis. Aspiration of blood from the joint is often necessary before a diagnosis can be made. With the knee flexed at 90°, the tibia is pulled forward on the femoral condyles. Forward displacement of more than 1 cm is a positive anterior drawer sign. The test is most sensitive, however, when compared with results on the normal side. Anterior displacement of greater than 0.5 cm over that of the normal side is consistent with a torn anterior cruciate ligament. The quality of the "end point" is also significant. A sudden, or "hard," stop suggests an intact ligament, whereas a "soft," less distinct end point is suggestive of a torn anterior cruciate ligament. The evaluation of the quality of the end point is quite subjective yet useful to experienced examiners in the testing of all ligaments about the knee. The posterior drawer test is performed in the same manner as the anterior drawer test except the tibia is pushed posteriorly. Posterior displacement of the tibia on the femur is suggestive of a ruptured posterior cruciate ligament. The Lachman test is also useful for testing the integrity of the anterior cruciate ligament. The patient is placed in the supine position with the knee in 15° of flexion. The examiner stabilizes the patient's distal thigh with one hand and grasps the patient's leg just distal to the tibiofemoral joint with the other hand. The examiner then attempts to move the tibia in an anterior direction. A soft end point and observable translation of the tibia relative to the normal side constitutes a positive test.

338. The answer is A. *(Morrissy, 4/e, p 71.)* Patients with Sprengel's deformity generally present at an early age. Sprengel's deformity is congenital elevation of the scapula, which causes the affected side of the neck to appear fuller and shorter. Affected patients may have limited abduction of the shoulder.

339. The answer is B. *(Evarts, 2/e, p 40.)* The signs and symptoms of fat embolism syndrome are those of adult respiratory distress syndrome in association with musculoskeletal trauma. The predominant feature is acute respiratory failure. Petechiae are found in 50 to 60 percent of cases, generally on the anterior chest and neck, axillae, and conjunctivae.

340. The answer is C. *(Rockwood, 4/e, pp 1213, 1247–1251.)* Most glenohumeral dislocations are anterior and usually result from forced abduction, extension, and external rotation. The head of the humerus usually lies anterior and inferior to the coracoid process. Early inspection will usually reveal flattening of the deltoid and the loss of the greater tuberosity as the most lateral point of the shoulder. When viewed from the front, the patient may have a prominent acromion process with a squared-off appearance of the shoulder. The patient is generally in severe pain and holds the dislocated arm in slight abduction and external rotation.

341. The answer is A. *(Sapira, p 424.)* Patients often present complaining of pain in an area other than the site of the pathologic process. For this reason, the "chief complaint" is often misleading. Pain originating at the hip joint is most often perceived in the groin area, followed by the buttock or posterior aspect of the greater trochanter. Occasionally pain may be referred to the ipsilateral knee.

342. The answer is B. *(Sapira, p 423.)* The crossed straight-leg raising test is performed with the patient in the supine position. The test is considered positive when straight-leg raising of the nonpainful leg worsens the pain on the other side. A positive test is indicative of disk herniation.

343–347. The answers are 343-D, 344-A, 345-B, 346-C, 347-E. *(Crenshaw, 8/e, pp 325–327, 2263–2267, 3108–3109, 3301–3339. Miller, 2/e, pp 47–48, 124–125, 431–450.)* The ulnar nerve is the terminal continuation of the medial cord of the brachial plexus and is composed of fibers from C8 and T1. It supplies no muscles in the arm, one and one-half muscles in the forearm, and most intrinsic muscles of the hand. Injuries of the lower brachial plexus or ulnar nerve are a common cause of clawhand. Clawhand is characterized by hyperextension of the metacarpophalangeal joints and flexion of the interphalangeal joints. When the intrinsic muscles are paralyzed, the unopposed long flexors of the fingers cause flexion of the interphalangeal joints of the fingers, and the unopposed long extensor muscles extend the metacarpophalangeal joints.

Achondroplasia is a physeal dysplasia that results in dwarfism. Inherited as an autosomal dominant trait, achondroplasia causes a decrease in the proliferation of cartilage in the growth plates. Appositional growth at the metaphysis is not affected, nor is intramembranous bone formation at the periosteum. This unbalanced growth of tubular bones results in the development of bones that are short and thick. Trident hands are characteristic of achondroplasia: the fingers are short and uniform in length and radiate out from the hand in a spokelike fashion.

Rheumatoid arthritis is a multisystem disease characterized by a chronic polyarthritis. The disease usually affects peripheral joints in a symmetric fashion. It is inflammatory in nature and characterized by cartilage destruction, bone erosion, and joint deformities. Inflammatory arthritis causes generalized stiffness that is usually worse after periods of rest. Morning stiffness of greater than 1 h in duration is characteristic. The characteristic joint deformities of the hand include radial deviation of the wrist, ulnar deviation of the digits at the metacarpophalangeal joints, hyperextension of the proximal interphalangeal joints and flexion of the distal interphalangeal joints (swan-neck deformity), and flexion of the proximal interphalangeal joints with extension of the distal interphalangeal joints (boutonnière deformity).

The radial nerve is a continuation of the posterior cord of the brachial plexus. It is composed of fibers from C6, C7, C8, and sometimes T1. It innervates the extensors of the elbow, wrist, fingers and thumb, and also the supinators of the forearm. Common causes of radial nerve paralysis include brachial plexus injuries, fractures of the humerus, and penetrating wounds of the arm and proximal forearm. A patient with radial nerve palsy will be unable to overcome gravitational pull and maintain wrist extension with the forearm in the pronated position. The wrist drops during this test ("wristdrop").

The median nerve is formed by the junction of the lateral and medial cords of the brachial plexus. It is composed of fibers from C6, C7, C8, and T1. The median nerve supplies no muscles in the arm, most flexors in the forearm, and five muscles in the hand, including the muscles of the thenar eminence. The recurrent branch of the median nerve innervates the thenar muscles. It lies superficially and may be damaged with superficial lacerations to this region. Long-standing paralysis of the median nerve by trauma or carpal tunnel syndrome results in thenar atrophy.

348–352. The answers are 348-A, 349-C, 350-B, 351-D, 352-E. (*Gartland, 4/e, pp 265, 267. Miller, 2/e, pp 246–248, 259–260, 267, 359, 361.*) Dupuytren's contracture is a fibrotic process of the palmar fascia that may affect one or both hands. The process most commonly causes fixed flexion of the ring finger and, to a lesser extent, the little finger. This process is often hereditary and may involve the soles of the feet and the corpora cavernosa of the penis (Peyronie's disease).

Most ganglia arise from joints of the wrist, but any joint or tendon sheath may give rise to ganglia. They may or may not be painful. Variation in size is a characteristic of ganglion cysts. They may or may not be fluctuant.

Mallet finger is generally the result of traumatic rupture of the extensor tendon of the distal phalanx. The unopposed flexor tendon holds the distal phalanx in flexion.

Carpal tunnel syndrome is the result of median nerve compression by the transverse carpal ligament. Patients experience numbness and tingling, which often worsens at night. Thenar atrophy and altered sensibility over the median nerve distribution may also occur. Positive symptoms of paresthesia or pain may be reproduced by percussion of the volar surface of the wrist (Tinel's sign) or by maintaining full flexion of the wrist for up to 1 min (Phalen's wrist flexion test).

Boxer's fracture is a frequently seen fracture through the neck of the fourth or fifth metacarpals. The head of the metacarpal is generally displaced toward the palm, which results in flattening of the knuckle prominence. As the name implies, this injury is usually a result of striking an object with the clenched fist.

353–357. The answers are 353-B, 354-D, 355-A, 356-E, 357-C. *(Gartland, 4/e, p 228. Miller, 2/e, pp 46–50, 188, 191, 371–374.)* Pain on abduction can accompany both bicipital and rotator cuff tendinitis. Bicipital tendinitis has a positive Yergason's sign, which is pain produced by supination of the forearm against resistance.

Circinate balanitis is a dermatitis of the glans penis. It is one of many possible cutaneous lesions associated with Reiter's syndrome. Along with cutaneous lesions, Reiter's syndrome classically involves the triad of conjunctivitis, urethritis, and arthritis.

Paralysis of the serratus anterior muscle (innervated by the long thoracic nerve) allows the scapula to protrude posteriorly from the posterior thoracic wall (winged scapula). This sign can be elicited by asking the patient to stand in front of and push against a wall.

Shoulder dislocation is usually anterior in nature and is associated with stretching or tearing of the subscapularis muscle and joint capsule. Affected patients may have a flattened shoulder profile and pain that is made worse with the use of the arm. The arm is usually held next to the trunk with the opposite extremity.

358–362. The answers are 358-A, 359-C, 360-B, 361-E, 362-D. *(Mann, Orthop Clin North Am 20:519–533, 1989. Sullivan, Clin Orthop 187:188, 1984.)* Improper shoe wear results in chronic pressure against the great toe, which may result in stretching of the capsular tissue along the medial aspect of the first metatarsophalangeal joint. This in turn results in a lateral deviation of the great toe (valgus deformity), which is accentuated by the laterally displaced extensor and flexor hallucis longus tendons. The patient's presenting complaint may be rubbing of the second toe or bunion formation. The second toe may be displaced superiorly by the laterally deviated great toe. A bunion may form on the medial aspect of the first metatarsophalangeal joint secondary to the hallux valgus deformity and shoe wear.

Swan-neck deformity is a common finger instability associated with rheumatoid arthritis. This deformity involves hyperextension of the proximal interphalangeal joint and flexion of the distal interphalangeal joint.

Hammer toe usually affects the second toe. The metatarsophalangeal joint is dorsiflexed and the proximal interphalangeal joint has plantar flexion. A painful corn may develop on the dorsum of the proximal interphalangeal joint from pressure on the shoe.

Stress fractures commonly occur in runners, particularly long-distance runners. The tibia is the most common site of stress fracture, followed by the metatarsal bones. The second and third metatarsals are most commonly involved. A stress fracture of a metatarsal is called a "march fracture." It is commonly seen in military recruits. Stress results in bone resorption followed by remodeling, i.e., the laying down of new bone along the lines of stress (Wolff's law). When sufficient time is not allowed for remodeling, prior to the onset of new stressors, stress fractures may occur. Radiographic findings are often not present; therefore, a good history and physical examination may be crucial to the proper diagnosis. Furthermore, a physician may be able to intervene when microfractures are present, remove the stress, and prevent the development of a complete fracture. Pertinent clues in the history include new activity, increase in activity, a change in running surface, or a change in shoes. Symptoms generally include pain with activity and relief during rest. The best sign is point tenderness, which may be associated with soft tissue swelling.

The primary manifestation of gout is a painful arthritis. Ninety-five percent of the cases are monarthric. Most of these occur in men and involve the metatarsophalangeal joint of the great toe. Many patients have a history of prior episodes.

363–367. The answers are 363-E, 364-C, 365-A, 366-B, 367-D. *(Crenshaw, 8/e, pp 1512–1514, 1963–1964, 1980–1981, 2008–2009, 2469.)* Muscular dystrophy is characterized by progressive weakness and muscular atrophy. Pseudohypertrophy may exist because of fatty infiltrates.

Osgood-Schlatter disease occurs in adolescence and is usually self-limiting. It is thought to be due to patellar tendon stress, which causes pain in the region of the tibial tuberosity. Physical findings include swelling and tenderness of the tibial tuberosity. Symptoms are reproduced by having the patient extend the knee against resistance.

Juvenile rheumatoid arthritis is an inflammatory disorder that begins in childhood and may produce extraarticular symptoms, including iridocyclitis, fever, rash, anemia, and pericarditis.

Rickets is generally attributed to vitamin D deficiency or renal malfunction and is manifested as bowing of the long bones, enlargement of the epiphyses of the long bones, delayed closure of the fontanels, and enlargement of the costochondral junctions of the ribs (rachitic rosary).

A patient with a torn meniscus of the knee may report symptoms of catching, snapping, clicking, locking, and giving way. The McMurray test may be useful in establishing the diagnosis. The patient is placed in the supine position with the knee fully flexed. The examiner holds the patient's foot in one hand and palpates the knee with the other hand. To check the medial meniscus, the leg is externally rotated and the knee is slowly extended. The examiner palpates the posteromedial margins of the joint for a palpable click as the femur passes over the torn meniscus. The lateral meniscus is tested by palpating the posterolateral margin of the joint with the leg in full internal rotation as the knee is extended.

368–372. The answers are 368-E, 369-A, 370-B, 371-C, 372-D. *(Magee, 2/e, pp 249–255. Miller, 2/e, pp 149–150.)* Ober's test is used to evaluate iliotibial band tension, which may be affected by contracture of the tensor fasciae latae. The test is conducted with the patient lying on his or her side. The leg is passively abducted and extended with the knee flexed to 90°. The test is positive if the hip remains abducted when the examiner slowly lowers the thigh.

Ortolani's test is used to identify congenital dislocation of the hip in an infant. This test results in reduction of a dislocated hip. The test is performed with the patient in the supine position with the hips flexed. The examiner holds the infant's legs with the thumbs against the inside of the knee and thigh and the fingers over the posterior aspect of the proximal femur. An anteriorly directed force is applied to the posterior aspect of the proximal femur as the hips are abducted and externally rotated. If the hip is dislocated, a "click" or "clunk" will be noted as the hip is reduced into the acetabulum. This test is valid only for the first few weeks after birth. The dislocated hip must be reducible in order to obtain a positive test.

Barlow's test is performed in a manner similar to that of the Ortolani's test except a posteriorly directed force is applied to the proximal femur. A positive Barlow's test results in dislocation of a reduced hip. This test is positive if the hip dislocates as a result of the posteriorly directed force and implies that the hip is unstable. A positive Barlow's test results when a hip that is appropriately seated in the acetabulum is dislocated, whereas a positive Ortolani's test indicates that a dislocated hip has been reduced into the acetabulum. Remember that the *O* in Ortolani means that the femoral head is *Out* of the acetabulum. Barlow's test is thought to be accurate in patients who are up to 6 months of age.

The telescoping test is performed with the patient supine with the hip and knee flexed to 90°. A posteriorly directed force is applied to the femur followed by an anteriorly directed force. Little movement will occur in the reduced hip. However, if the hip is dislocated, a greater amount of translation is allowed because the head of the femur is not locked into the acetabulum.

Allis' test (Galeazzi's sign) is performed with the patient supine with the hips flexed to 90° and the knees fully flexed. The test is positive when one knee is higher than the other. This is an indication of relative femur length. A positive test may indicate a dislocated hip or a discrepancy in femur length.

373–374. The answers are 373-A, C; 374-F, G. *(Miller, 2/e, pp 257–259. Munro, 9/e, pp 290–296.)* Patients with rheumatoid arthritis may develop tenosynovitis. Flexor tenosynovitis can cause an accumulation of synovial tissue in the carpal tunnel. This may result in median nerve compression (carpal tunnel syndrome). Pain or numbness and tingling in the distribution of the median nerve (thumb, index, long, and radial half of ring fingers) suggest the diagnosis of carpal tunnel syndrome. Flexor tenosynovitis can cause enlargement of the flexor tendon sheaths where they pass through the pulleys of the digits. This causes a locking, or catching, as this enlarged portion of the tendon passes through the pulley. This condition is called *trigger finger* and is also common in patients with rheumatoid arthritis. Patients with rheumatoid arthritis often develop extensor tenosynovitis. This process can result in extensor tendon rupture. A patient with rupture of the extensor digitorum to the small finger and extensor digiti minimi tendons will be unable to extend the small finger. If only the latter is ruptured, lack of extension will only be present if the function of the extensor digitorum muscle is blocked by holding the other digits in flexion. Subluxation of the extensor tendon off of the dorsum of the MCP joint and into the valley between the metacarpal heads will result in an inability to obtain extension of the MCP joint. However, the patient will be able to maintain extension once the MCP joint is placed into extension. The tenodesis effect is an important part of the examination for patients with possible tendon rupture. When the wrist is passively flexed, the extensor tendons pull the fingers into extension. When the wrist is passively extended, the flexor tendons pull the fingers into flexion. The tenodesis effect is present with nerve injuries and lost with tendon ruptures. Patients with a ruptured extensor pollicis longus tendon are unable to lift the thumb up when the hand is placed palm down on a table.

375–377. The answers are 375-C, 376-B, 377-D. *(Crenshaw, 8/e, pp 3753–3756.)* The straight-leg raising test is performed with the patient in the supine position. The leg is slowly passively elevated while the knee is kept fully extended. The leg can normally be elevated up to 90° without much discomfort. Pain that radiates down the leg or into the feet, the back, or opposite side indicates nonspecific irritation of the sciatic nerve or roots. A pulling or tight sensation in the hamstring is often present and is *not* a positive test. If the knee is bent, which relaxes the sciatic nerve, the pain will often be relieved. Bending the knee has no effect on pain caused by disorders of the hip joint. After the straight-leg raising test has produced pain, dorsiflexion of the foot (Lasègue's sign) aggravates pain caused by irritation of the sciatic nerve. Active elevation of the leg causes a significant load across the hip joint and results in pain if arthritis of the hip joint is present (Stinchfield test).

378–379. The answers are 378-B, 379-A. *(Lewis, p 152.)* The tendons of the flexor digitorum profundus muscle insert on the bases of the distal phalanges of digits II through V. This muscle flexes all joints of the fingers, but is the only muscle to flex the distal interphalangeal joint. Isolating the distal interphalangeal joint allows the examiner to test the integrity of this muscle and tendon. The tendons of the flexor digitorum superficialis muscle insert on the shafts of the middle phalanges of digits II through V. By holding the uninvolved digits in full extension, the examiner locks the profundus muscle in the extended position to eliminate its action on the involved finger and isolates the superficialis tendon function.

Genitourinary System

DIRECTIONS: Each item below contains a question or incomplete statement followed by suggested responses. Select the **one best** response to each question.

380. As you are performing the external portion of the pelvic examination, you palpate a mass that is unilateral in the posterolateral portion of the labia majora. The patient notes that palpation is painful. The most likely diagnosis is

(A) Bartholin's cyst
(B) Bartholin's gland abscess
(C) Skene's cyst
(D) Skene's gland abscess
(E) rectocele

381. While examining the male genitalia, you are unable to retract the foreskin of an uncircumcised patient. There is no evidence of erythema. This condition is known as

(A) balanitis
(B) phimosis
(C) escutcheon
(D) smegma
(E) priapism

382. A 34-year-old man complains of lumps in his scrotal skin. The lumps are found to be small and mobile, and an oily material can be extruded from them. The most likely diagnosis is

(A) scrotal rings
(B) microcarcinoma of the scrotal type
(C) epidermoid cysts
(D) molluscum contagiosum
(E) condyloma acuminatum

383. A man complains of soft, raised, reddish lesions on his glans penis, prepuce, and penile shaft. Several excisional biopsies are done to look for possible malignant change. The most likely diagnosis is

(A) lymphogranuloma venereum
(B) Peyronie's disease
(C) condyloma acuminatum
(D) molluscum contagiosum
(E) syphilitic chancre

384. A 4-month-old child is brought to the emergency room. The parents have noted that the child's scrotum is enlarged. The physician found the mass nontender, smooth, and firm. The scrotum was distended but not taut. Using his penlight, he determined that the mass transilluminated. The most likely diagnosis is

(A) scrotal carcinoma
(B) spermatocele
(C) varicocele
(D) hydrocele
(E) epididymitis

385. A 21-year-old man who recently suffered through the mumps now presents to his physician complaining of a swollen and painful left testicle. The most likely diagnosis is

(A) orchitis
(B) epididymitis
(C) testicular tumor
(D) varicocele
(E) spermatocele

386. A 12-year-old boy presents with a 3-h history of a painful scrotum. Examination reveals an enlarged, tender, erythematous scrotum. The scrotum does not transilluminate, and the testicle is in a transverse lie. The most likely diagnosis is

(A) spermatocele
(B) hydrocele
(C) epididymitis
(D) varicocele
(E) testicular torsion

387. Choose the correct statement concerning digital rectal examination (DRE) and serum prostate-specific antigen (PSA) in the detection of prostate cancer.

(A) The combined use of DRE and PSA affords a more complete evaluation than either test alone
(B) DRE is more sensitive than PSA
(C) Neither DRE nor PSA is effective
(D) Either DRE or PSA allows complete assessment
(E) PSA should not be used for detection of prostate cancer

388. A 16-year-old patient presents to the emergency room with extreme penile pain. The ER physician notes that this uncircumcised patient has his foreskin retracted and that his glans penis is enlarged and bluish in color. The patient suffers extreme pain when the physician attempts to reposition the foreskin. The most likely diagnosis is

(A) hypospadias
(B) balanitis
(C) priapism
(D) paraphimosis
(E) phimosis

389. A 14-year-old boy complains of the gradual worsening of scrotal swelling and pain. He also complains of dysuria. On examination you note an edematous and erythematous scrotum. When you elevate the testicle, he feels much relief of his pain. The most likely diagnosis is

(A) orchitis
(B) epididymitis
(C) testicular torsion
(D) varicocele
(E) hydrocele

390. The vulva includes all the following EXCEPT

(A) labia majora
(B) labia minora
(C) clitoris
(D) hymen
(E) mons pubis

391. A 15-year-old boy complains of worsening scrotal pain. On palpation you find a pea-sized, tender mass at the upper pole of the testis. With transillumination it appears as a "blue dot." The most likely diagnosis is

(A) testicular torsion
(B) epididymitis
(C) hernia with hydrocele
(D) appendix testis torsion
(E) orchitis with hydrocele

392. A 24-year-old woman presents to her family physician with the chief complaint of having had no menstruation for the last 2 months. While the pregnancy test is being performed, the physician might find other signs of pregnancy, including all the following EXCEPT

(A) a bluish color to the cervix
(B) exaggerated uterine ante-flexion
(C) increased vaginal secretions
(D) striae radiating from the mons pubis
(E) tender breasts

393. Which of the following is associated with menopause?

(A) Pubic hair turns gray
(B) The vaginal introitus broadens
(C) The labia enlarge
(D) The vagina widens and has increased rugosity
(E) Vaginal secretions become more viscous

394. A 13-year-old boy is complaining of heaviness to his scrotum and a vague pain. He states that the pain is worsened by exertion. On palpation you feel dilated veins ("bag of worms") above his left testis. The most likely diagnosis is

(A) orchitis
(B) testicular torsion
(C) epididymitis
(D) varicocele
(E) hematocele

395. An 18-year-old man presents with a mass in the right inguinal area. When the physician digitally examines for herniation, she notes that when the patient coughs she feels a mass striking the lateral aspect of her examining finger. When she compresses the right inguinal area over the internal ring and again asks the patient to cough, her examining finger does not sense any mass striking it. Which of the following statements is true?

(A)   This type of hernia almost always resolves spontaneously before puberty

(B)   If the hernial sac extends into the scrotum, then this is a true surgical emergency

(C)   Inguinal hernias are more common in women

(D)   The appendix may be found in the hernial sac

(E)   This type of hernia is frequently present in elderly women

396. A 22-year-old man presents 1 day after having been a restrained driver involved in a moderate speed automobile accident. He is complaining only of a discolored (blue) scrotum. There was no trauma to the scrotum. You note that the discoloration is gravity-dependent. The most likely diagnosis is

(A)   fat necrosis
(B)   testicular torsion
(C)   inguinal hernia
(D)   hematocele
(E)   hydrocele

397. A 9-year-old girl is brought to your office by her mother, who states that the daughter has been losing weight and having difficulty at school. The mother discovered some yellow discharge on the child's underwear. On examination you note erythema to almost all parts of the vulva and to the vagina. There is a yellow discharge, The most likely diagnosis is

(A)   müllerian duct tumor
(B)   wolffian duct tumor
(C)   bubble-bath vaginitis
(D)   sexual abuse
(E)   straddle injury

398. Nocturia may be due to all the following EXCEPT

(A)   coffee
(B)   atropine
(C)   alcohol
(D)   congestive heart failure
(E)   nephrotic syndrome

399. All the following statements regarding scrotal anatomy are correct EXCEPT

(A)   the softer, comma-shaped epididymis is situated on the posteromedial aspect of each testis

(B)   the left testis usually lies somewhat lower than the right

(C)   the epididymis is most prominent along the superior margin of the testis

(D)   a normal testis may range in length from 3.5 cm to 5.5 cm

(E)   the tunica vaginalis does not surround the posterior aspect of the testis

400. Which of the following statements regarding lymphatics is true?

(A) Lymphatics from the penile surfaces drain into the abdominal nodes

(B) Lymphatics from the scrotal surfaces drain into the abdominal nodes

(C) Lymphatics from the testes drain into the abdominal nodes

(D) Lymphatics from the testes drain into the inguinal nodes

(E) Penile and scrotal skin are without lymphatics

401. Which of the following is NOT typical of ureteral pain?

(A) Dull, aching pain

(B) Severe, colicky pain

(C) Possible radiation toward the umbilicus

(D) Possible radiation to the testicle or labium

(E) Nausea

402. Multiple, painful vesicles on the glans penis of a sexually active young patient would most likely indicate

(A) epispadias

(B) syphilis

(C) herpes genitalis (progenitalis)

(D) condylomata acuminata

(E) gonorrhea

DIRECTIONS: Each group of questions below consists of lettered options followed by numbered items. For each numbered item, select the appropriate lettered option(s). Each lettered option may be used once, more than once, or not at all. **Choose exactly the number of options indicated following each item.**

Items 403–405

Match the diagnostic findings on microscopic examination with the responsible organism.

(A) *Trichomonas vaginalis*
(B) *Neisseria gonorrhoeae*
(C) *Gardnerella vaginalis*
(D) *Staphylococcus vaginalis*
(E) *Candida albicans*

403. A pear-shaped organism on wet preparation **(SELECT 1 ORGANISM)**

404. Clue cells on wet preparation **(SELECT 1 ORGANISM)**

405. Hyphae with a potassium hydroxide (KOH) preparation **(SELECT 1 ORGANISM)**

Items 406–410

Match the diagnoses below with the appropriate findings.

(A) Firm, painless ulcer
(B) Imperforate hymen
(C) Shiny, red, friable tissue
(D) Protrusion of posterior vaginal wall
(E) Protrusion of anterior vaginal wall

406. Rectocele **(SELECT 1 FINDING)**

407. Cystocele **(SELECT 1 FINDING)**

408. Hydrocolpos **(SELECT 1 FINDING)**

409. Ectropion **(SELECT 1 FINDING)**

410. Chancre **(SELECT 1 FINDING)**

DIRECTIONS: Each group of questions below consists of four lettered options followed by a set of numbered items. For each numbered item select

A	if the item is associated with	(A) only
B	if the item is associated with	(B) only
C	if the item is associated with	**both** (A) and (B)
D	if the item is associated with	**neither** (A) nor (B)

Each lettered option may be used **once, more than once, or not at all.**

Items 411–415

   (A) Prostatitis
   (B) Cystitis
   (C) Both
   (D) Neither

411. Urinary urgency

412. Dysuria

413. Hesitancy in starting the urinary stream

414. Reduced force of urinary stream

415. Hematuria

Genitourinary System

Answers

380. The answer is B. *(Seidel, 3/e, pp 586, 637.)* Abscesses are generally painful to palpation, hot to the touch, and fluctuant. The abscess is usually gonococcal or staphylococcal in origin and is filled with pus. A rectocele is a bulging mass that is present on the posterior wall of the vagina. It represents a weakness in the investing fascia of the posterior vaginal wall.

381. The answer is B. *(Seidel, 3/e, pp 604–605.)* Phimosis is the condition in which the foreskin in an uncircumcised patient cannot be retracted; this may occur normally during the first 6 years of life. Phimosis is usually congenital, but may be due to recurrent infections or balanoposthitis (inflammation of the glans penis and prepuce). Balanitis is inflammation of the glans penis and occurs only in uncircumcised persons. Escutcheon is the hair pattern associated with the genitalia. Smegma is a white, cheesy material that collects around the glans penis in an uncircumcised patient. Priapism is a prolonged penile erection, which is often painful.

382. The answer is C. *(Seidel, 3/e, pp 605–609, 616–621.)* Epidermoid, or sebaceous, cysts appear as small lumps in the scrotal skin, which may enlarge and discharge oily material. Molluscum contagiosum is caused by a poxvirus and is sexually transmitted. The lesions are smooth and dome-shaped with discrete margins and occur most commonly on the glans penis.

383. The answer is C. *(Seidel, 3/e, pp 584, 616, 618.)* Lymphogranuloma venereum is a sexually transmitted disease caused by a chlamydial organism. It initially presents as painless erosions and later may involve the lymphatics. Peyronie's disease is unilateral deviation of the penis caused by a fibrous band in the corpus cavernosum. A syphilitic chancre is painless, with indurated borders and a clear base appearing 2 weeks after exposure. Scrapings from the chancre will reveal spirochetes. Condyloma acuminatum, or venereal warts, are caused by the human papillomavirus (HPV). They occur on skin and mucosal surfaces of external genitalia and perianal areas. They are sexually transmitted, with an incubation period of 1 to 6 months. The lesions are soft, pink-to-red growths on various parts of the penis and can undergo malignant degeneration.

384. The answer is D. *(Seidel, 3/e, pp 618–620.)* Hydrocele is common in infancy, and if the tunica vaginalis is not patent, the hydrocele will usually resolve during the first 6 months of life. A spermatocele does transilluminate, but it does not grow as large as a hydrocele and remains localized as a cystic swelling on the epididymis. A varicocele is due to torsion of the pampiniform plexus that surrounds the spermatic cord. It usually occurs on the left side in boys or young men and can be quite painful. Epididymitis occurs most frequently in association with urinary tract infections and is very painful. The scrotum may be tense and is usually quite erythematous. Epididymitis can mimic testicular torsion, a surgical emergency.

385. The answer is A. *(Seidel, 3/e, pp 605–619.)* Orchitis is an uncommon occurrence except as a sequela of infection with mumps in young males. It is most often unilateral and testicular atrophy occurs in 50 percent of cases. Testicular tumors are the most common neoplasm in men 15 to 30 years of age. The tumors do not transilluminate, they are not tender, they are fixed to the testicle, and most are malignant. Epididymitis presents as an enlarged, very erythematous, extremely tender scrotum and is usually associated with a urinary tract infection. A varicocele is usually a left-sided swelling of the scrotal sac, which when palpated feels like "a bag of worms." A spermatocele is a swelling of the epididymis; it does transilluminate, but remains localized to the epididymis.

386. The answer is E. *(McCullough, pp 24–25.)* The tunica vaginalis normally attaches the posterolateral surfaces of the testicle to the scrotum, thereby anchoring it and preventing rotation. When these attachments are missing, the testicle is free to rotate around the spermatic cord and the critical vascular pedicle. This is known as *intravaginal torsion* and is most common in patients 10 to 19 years of age. Classically, the testicle will have a transverse lie within the scrotum, known as the "bell-clapper" relationship. Onset of pain is sudden and there are no urinary complaints. Many feel that the initiating factor may be contraction of the cremaster muscle. Loss of cremasteric reflex is almost invariably found in torsion.

387. The answer is A. *(Yamamoto, Int J Urol 1:74, 1994.)* Serum PSA measurement is more reliable than DRE for detection of prostate cancer. Since these two methods do not always detect the same malignancy, the combined use of DRE and PSA affords a more complete evaluation for detecting prostate cancer.

388. The answer is D. *(Seidel, 3/e, pp 604–616.)* Hypospadias is a congenital abnormality in which the urethra is situated on the ventral surface of the shaft of the penis. Balanitis can occur in an uncircumcised man and is an inflammation of the glans penis. Priapism is a painful, long-standing erection that most often occurs in patients with leukemia or sickle cell anemia. Paraphimosis is a condition that occurs when the foreskin cannot be returned to the extended position; it may lead to gangrene of the glans penis. Phimosis is the inability to retract the foreskin.

389. The answer is B. *(McCullough, pp 24–28.)* Epididymitis in children usually occurs in the preteenage years and is thought to be most often due to reflux of sterile urine that causes an inflammatory reaction in the epididymis. A urinary tract infection is occasionally seen. There is tenderness of the posterolaterally positioned epididymis with a normal testicle palpated anteriorly. When the testicle is elevated and the patient experiences relief from pain this is known as Prehn's sign. This sign is unreliable, and testicular torsion always needs to be ruled out.

390. The answer is D. *(Seidel, 3/e, pp 530–531.)* The vulva, also known as the external female genital organs, includes the mons pubis (veneris), labia majora, labia minora, clitoris, vestibular glands, vaginal vestibule, and urethral opening. The hymen is more internal and surrounds the vaginal opening. The hymen is a connective tissue membrane that separates the vestibule of the vagina from the vagina proper. Once perforated, only a ring or hymenal tags remain.

391. The answer is D. *(McCullough, pp 26–27.)* There are two intrascrotal appendages that may suffer torsion. The appendix testis and the appendix epididymidis are embryonic ductal system remnants. Torsion can occur at any time, but the peak occurrence is between the ages of 10 and 15 years. Onset of pain can be sudden or gradual. The infarcted appendage can often be seen as a "blue dot" on the superior pole of the testis. Reactive hydrocele or scrotal erythema may mask the blue dot, whereas transillumination may highlight its appearance.

392. The answer is D. *(Seidel, 3/e, pp 161–162, 536–537.)* There is increased blood flow to the uterus, the cervix, and the isthmus during pregnancy, and an associated increase in lymphatic flow, which causes pelvic congestion and an edematous condition. The cervix will appear bluish, and with compression of the isthmus by the edema there is exaggerated uterine anteflexion during the first 3 months of the pregnancy. The most common symptoms in the early months of pregnancy are amenorrhea, urinary frequency, breast enlargement, tender breasts, nausea, and easy fatigability. The hormonal changes cause an increase in vaginal secretions. Striae radiating from around the umbilicus occur late in pregnancy as a result of the increasing size of the uterus.

393. The answer is A. *(Seidel, 3/e, pp 538, 710.)* Menstrual periods cease sometime between 40 and 55 years of age, and this is only one aspect of the transitional phase of the life cycle known as menopause. With the decreased estrogen at this time the size of the labia and the clitoris decreases, the labia flatten owing to loss of fat, pubic hair becomes more sparse and turns gray, the vaginal introitus constricts, and the vagina narrows, shortens, and loses its rugosity. The vaginal mucosa becomes thin, pale, and dry. The uterus decreases in size, the endometrium thins, the cervix becomes small and pale, and the ovaries decrease in size to approximately 1 to 2 cm. Approximately three-fourths of menopausal women experience hot flashes. Osteoporosis is an important health hazard in postmenopausal women. It is characterized by a reduction in the quantity of bone, which increases the incidence of fractures.

394. The answer is D. *(McCullough, p 29.)* Varicocele is dilated veins of the pampiniform plexus. The incidence is rare before 8 years of age, and a plateau is reached at puberty. The cause is venous stasis and reflux into the spermatic vein, which is due to compression of the left renal vein at the level of the aorta. The dilated veins, or "bag of worms," are more easily seen and palpated with the patient standing. Retroperitoneal disease needs to be excluded, and if the testis is diminished in size, then surgery is indicated in an attempt to preserve fertility.

395. The answer is D. *(Seidel, 3/e, pp 606–615.)* All hernias except femoral hernias are more common in males. Most hernias are not surgical emergencies. Hernias are surgical emergencies if they are incarcerated, which is when the hernial sac is irreducible. When it has compromised circulation, it is known as strangulated. The appendix, or any other visceral organ, may be found within the hernial sac.

396. The answer is D. *(McCullough, pp 33–34.)* The presence of a patent processus vaginalis allows communication of intraperitoneal contents with the scrotum. Clear intraperitoneal fluid can form a hydrocele. Purulent material from a ruptured appendix can cause a hot scrotum. There have been unusual cases of scrotal swelling due to meconium in the newborn and due to migration of ventriculoperitoneal shunt tubing. Abdominal trauma, as from a seat belt, can disrupt intraabdominal contents, and the blood can migrate through a patent processus vaginalis. The scrotal blood will not transilluminate and it may be gravity-dependent.

397. The answer is D. *(Bates, 5/e, pp 485–486.)* Speculum examination of a school-aged child must be performed by an experienced practitioner and should be done with the same respect given the adult woman. Swelling and erythema of vulvar tissue should be a "red flag" for child abuse, especially if associated with bruising or a foul-smelling discharge. A sexually transmitted disease would seem pathognomonic. In addition to the anorectal and genitourinary problems, there can be significant behavioral changes, such as sexually provocative mannerisms, excessive masturbation, inappropriate sexual knowledge, depression, school problems, and weight changes. A straddle injury from a bicycle seat occurs over the symphysis pubis, whereas signs of sexual abuse are more posterior around the perineum. Bubble-bath vaginitis is not uncommon and does not require a speculum examination.

398. The answer is B. *(Bates, 5/e, pp 54, 85.)* Nocturia can be classified into high-volume output or low-volume output. Low-volume nocturia (frequency without polyuria) can be caused by cystitis, bladder stones, upper motor neuron disease, prostatic hypertrophy, or anxiety. Insomnia can also result in nocturia, which occurs while the patient is up yet has no real urge to void; this is called "pseudofrequency." Nocturia with high-volume output can be caused by excessive coffee or alcohol intake just prior to bedtime, congestive heart failure, nephrotic syndrome, hepatic cirrhosis with ascites, and chronic venous insufficiency. Atropine is an anticholinergic and thus would cause an increase in urethral sphincter tone with attendant difficulty with urinary flow, not nocturia.

399. The answer is A. *(Bates, 5/e, pp 369–381.)* The epididymis is generally situated on the posterolateral aspect of the testis, though it may be located anteriorly in 6 to 7 percent of males. It consists of three subdivisions: head, body, and tail. The duct of the epididymis is continuous with the ductus deferens.

400. The answer is C. *(Bates, 5/e, p 370.)* The lymphatics from both the penile and the scrotal surfaces drain into the inguinal nodes; thus, when you find inflammation on these surfaces, you must assess the inguinal nodes for enlargement and tenderness. The lymphatics from the testes drain into the abdominal nodes and when enlarged are not accessible by physical examination.

401. The answer is A. *(Bates, 5/e, p 53.)* When there is disease in the kidney or the ureter, the pain can be in the back or the abdomen. Kidney pain is classically elicited by percussion at the costovertebral angle (CVA). It is a visceral type of pain that is due to distention of the renal capsule, and it is typically dull, aching, and steady. Ureteral colic, or extension of this process into the renal pelvis, is a distinctly different type of pain than kidney pain. It is a severe, colicky pain that usually begins at the costovertebral angle and can radiate around to the abdomen and extend into the testicle or the labium. Ureteral colic is most often caused by a sudden obstruction of the ureter by urinary calculi.

402. The answer is C. *(Isselbacher, 13/e, pp 534–543.)* The syphilitic chancre, like the condylomata, is generally a painless lesion. Gonorrhea in the male is characterized by purulent urethral discharge rather than lesions on the external genitalia. Epispadias is a congenital defect in which the urethral meatus appears on the dorsum of the penis.

403–405. The answers are 403-A, 404-C, 405-E. *(Seidel, 3/e, pp 583–584, 587.)* Even before obtaining the vaginal secretions, you should prepare the appropriate glass slides. If you suspect *Gardnerella vaginalis*, a wet-preparation slide is used, and clue cells will be diagnostic. Clue cells are epithelial cells with adherent bacteria that cause their border to be irregular. *Gardnerella* infection commonly causes a very profuse, malodorous discharge.

For detection of *Trichomonas vaginalis*, the vaginal secretions, which are usually a frothy, yellow-green or gray, are mixed with one drop of saline solution on the glass slide, and diagnosis is made after observing motile, pear-shaped organisms. Ten percent of patients affected with *Trichomonas* will also have petechiae, known as strawberry patches, on their cervix or vaginal mucosa.

For detection of *Candida albicans,* the vaginal secretions, which have a cottage-cheese appearance, are mixed on a glass slide that has a drop of potassium hydroxide (KOH) solution. Diagnosis is made by the appearance of hyphae, which may also have budding present. *Candida* infection causes the patient much discomfort from vulvar itching and burning.

406–410. The answers are 406-D, 407-E, 408-B, 409-C, 410-A. *(Seidel, 3/e, pp 584–589.)* A rectocele is a protrusion of a part of the rectum through the posterior vaginal wall. Examination is enhanced by having the patient bear down. A rectocele is also known as a proctocele.

A cystocele is the protrusion of the urinary bladder through the anterior vaginal wall. Examination can again be aided by having the patient bear down. In severe cases, the bladder may protrude through the introitus and may have attendant urinary stress incontinence.

Hydrocolpos is a collection of vaginal secretions behind an imperforate hymen. Hematocolpos is a collection of blood in the vaginal vault that is common in menarche when there is an imperforate hymen.

Ectropion is columnar epithelium from the cervical canal and is shiny and red in appearance. Ectropion is not a pathologic finding, but it may bleed easily when examined, and a Pap smear or biopsy should be performed to rule out cervical carcinoma.

A syphilitic chancre, found in primary syphilis, is a firm, painless ulcer. Chancres in women are usually undetected because they are located internally.

411–415. The answers are 411-B, 412-C, 413-A, 414-A, 415-B. *(Bates, 5/e, pp 53–55.)* Prostatitis is inflammation of the prostate gland, and the pain is usually felt in the perineum and occasionally in the rectum. When the prostate is enlarged there will be at least some obstruction, and this can manifest with a group of symptoms: hesitancy in starting the urinary stream, straining to void, reduced caliber and force of the urinary stream, and dribbling of urine after the patient attempts to stop urinating. *Dysuria* is often used, narrowly, to mean pain upon urination, but many clinicians use the term to mean any abnormality with urination. Cystitis is inflammation of the bladder, and this causes irritation of the bladder that stimulates the detrusor muscle to contract and leads to the urge to void, i.e., urinary urgency. This condition sometimes leads to urge incontinence. Whenever urge incontinence is present, it represents pathology most often in the bladder, but it could indicate disorder in the urethra, in the surrounding structures, or in the neural regulatory mechanisms that control urination.

Dermatology

DIRECTIONS: Each item below contains a question or incomplete statement followed by suggested responses. Select the **one best** response to each question.

416. A patient presents with severe pruritus that is worse at night and reports similar symptoms among other family members. Upon examination, areas of excoriated papules are observed in the interdigital area. This history is most consistent with the diagnosis of

(A) dermatitis herpetiformis
(B) cutaneous larva migrans
(C) contact dermatitis
(D) scabies
(E) impetigo

417. A 6-year-old child presents complaining of patchy hair loss on the back of the scalp. Examination reveals well-demarcated areas of erythema and scaling, and although there is still some hair in the area, it is noted that the hairs are extremely short and broken in appearance. The patient is most likely suffering from

(A) cutaneous candidiasis
(B) tinea capitis
(C) androgenic hair loss
(D) scalp psoriasis
(E) seborrheic dermatitis

418. A 20-year-old woman presents with a 2-week history of 1- to 3-cm areas of scaly plaques on the knees and trunk. They are noted to be pruritic, and upon examination, there are erythematous lesions with small bleeding points when scraped (Auspitz's sign). The patient is suffering from

(A) Kaposi's sarcoma
(B) pemphigus
(C) psoriasis
(D) systemic lupus erythematosus (SLE)
(E) hairy leukoplakia

419. Features characteristic of cutaneous malignancies include all the following EXCEPT

(A) frequent association with sun exposure
(B) ulcerated surface
(C) poorly defined borders
(D) variable pigmentation
(E) lesions of 3 to 5 mm in diameter

420. A 10-year-old child presents with vesicular lesions on the hands and face, some of which have ruptured and expressed a serous exudate. A Tzanck preparation is negative for multinucleated giant cells, but Gram stain shows gram-positive cocci. The most likely diagnosis is

(A)   cellulitis
(B)   folliculitis
(C)   impetigo
(D)   Kawasaki's disease
(E)   staphylococcal scalded-skin syndrome

421. A 37-year-old man who works in a fish market presents with a burning pain in his right hand of 1 week's duration. Physical examination reveals a large, violaceous plaque on his finger. Gram stain reveals no organism. The likely diagnosis is

(A)   erythrasma
(B)   erysipeloid
(C)   ecthyma
(D)   erysipelas
(E)   purpura

422. A patient presents with painless papules that arose following a puncture wound from a rose thorn a few weeks earlier. Physical examination reveals a chain of erythematous nodules along the dorsal aspect of the arm. The most likely diagnosis is

(A)   *Candida albicans* infection
(B)   blastomycosis
(C)   tinea versicolor
(D)   sporotrichosis
(E)   cutaneous larva migrans

423. All the following statements are true of herpes zoster EXCEPT

(A)   it is due to a reactivation of latent varicella virus
(B)   erupted lesions usually involve a single dermatome
(C)   it is limited to adults
(D)   it is usually more severe in the immunocompromised person
(E)   it is typically very painful

424. A child presents complaining of multiple bumps on the hand. Examination reveals lesions that are approximately 4 mm in diameter and have a central umbilication and erythematous base. This is most likely

(A)   due to a varicella virus
(B)   milker's nodule
(C)   rubeola
(D)   erythema infectiosum
(E)   molluscum contagiosum

425. All the following statements are true concerning nummular eczema EXCEPT

(A)   exacerbations are associated with dry skin
(B)   it may be exacerbated by emotional factors
(C)   it occurs in all age groups
(D)   it is very seldom pruritic
(E)   it is often associated with an atopic family history

426. All the following statements are true of capillary hemangiomas EXCEPT

(A) they are most commonly found on the head
(B) they can become large and very alarming
(C) surgery is usually necessary
(D) they usually present as a small, red nodule
(E) they can be easily susceptible to bleeding

427. Staphylococcal scalded-skin syndrome (SSSS) may be characterized by all the following statements EXCEPT

(A) it is associated with pharyngitis and conjunctivitis
(B) it occurs only in infants
(C) bullous lesions result in a positive Nikolsky's sign
(D) once healed, there is usually no severe scarring
(E) lesions are the result of a bacterial toxin

428. Cutaneous manifestations of bacterial endocarditis include all the following EXCEPT

(A) subconjunctival hemorrhage
(B) Janeway's lesions
(C) Osler's nodes
(D) splinter hemorrhages
(E) spider angiomas

429. All the following are true statements regarding porphyria cutanea tarda EXCEPT

(A) it is the most common form of porphyria in the U.S.
(B) ethanol and estrogen therapy are considered to be important precipitating agents
(C) it demonstrates autosomal recessive inheritance
(D) lesions occur on sun-exposed areas
(E) increased hair (hypertrichosis) on the face and arms is a manifestation

430. All the following statements concerning lichen planus are true EXCEPT

(A) lesions typically occur on the flexor aspects of the wrists and ankles, the penis, and oral mucous membranes
(B) it occurs more commonly in males
(C) lesions appear as flat-topped papules with numerous white lines (Wickham's striae)
(D) it is of unknown etiology
(E) lesions can occur locally or be widespread

431. Lyme disease is correctly described by all the following statements EXCEPT

(A) lesions are annular in appearance with firm, bluish-red borders
(B) arthritis may develop
(C) the causative agent is *Borrelia burgdorferi*
(D) the disease often presents as a solitary lesion that enlarges over a period of several days
(E) the patient can usually associate the lesion with a tick bite

432. All the following are associated with measles EXCEPT

(A) otitis media and bronchopneumonia
(B) a prodrome that includes conjunctivitis, cough, and fever
(C) upward progression of an erythematous, maculopapular rash
(D) oral lesions appearing as blue-white spots on erythematous bases (Koplik's spots)
(E) viral etiology

433. A 43-year-old woman presents with large hands, a large mandible, and coarse, leathery facial skin. The most likely diagnosis is

(A) Marfan's syndrome
(B) hypothyroidism
(C) scleroderma
(D) acromegaly
(E) Cushing's syndrome

434. A 40-year-old woman presents with puffiness around the eyes, brittle hair, coarse skin, and complaints of fatigue and cold intolerance. The most likely diagnosis is

(A) hypothyroidism
(B) hyperthyroidism
(C) congestive heart failure
(D) Cushing's disease
(E) nephrotic syndrome

435. A 13-year-old boy who has just recovered from the "flu" presents with lethargy, vomiting, delirium, and hepatomegaly. The most likely diagnosis is

(A) Reye's syndrome
(B) St. Louis encephalitis
(C) viral hepatitis
(D) salicylate toxicity
(E) Wilson's disease

436. A 4-year-old child is brought in by her mother because of a painful, honey-colored, crusted lesion on her face. The most likely diagnosis is

(A) miliaria
(B) impetigo
(C) cellulitis
(D) seborrheic dermatitis
(E) chickenpox

DIRECTIONS: Each group of questions below consists of lettered options followed by numbered items. For each numbered item, select the appropriate lettered option(s). Each lettered option may be used once, more than once, or not at all. **Choose exactly the number of options indicated following each item.**

Items 437–441

Match each of the nail manifestations below with the appropriate disease.

(A) Psoriasis
(B) Hepatic cirrhosis
(C) Iron deficiency anemia
(D) Renal disease and azotemia
(E) Respiratory disease

437. Koilonychia **(SELECT 1 DISEASE)**

438. White nails with only the distal 1 to 2 mm pink **(SELECT 1 DISEASE)**

439. Nails that are white on the proximal half and pink or brown on the distal half **(SELECT 1 DISEASE)**

440. Pitting **(SELECT 1 DISEASE)**

441. Clubbing **(SELECT 1 DISEASE)**

Items 442–445

Match each description with the appropriate type of hair loss.

(A) Telogen effluvium
(B) Androgenetic hair loss
(C) Alopecia areata
(D) Alopecia universalis
(E) Trichotillomania

442. Smooth, circumscribed patches of hair loss **(SELECT 1 TYPE)**

443. Occurrence in postpartum period **(SELECT 1 TYPE)**

444. Frontotemporal recession **(SELECT 1 TYPE)**

445. Psychological disturbance **(SELECT 2 TYPES)**

Items 446–450

Match each factor with the appropriate disease.

(A) Acrodermatitis enteropathica
(B) Dermatomyositis
(C) Pityriasis rosea
(D) Chancroid
(E) von Recklinghausen's disease

446. "Christmas tree" pattern of lesions **(SELECT 1 DISEASE)**

447. Gram-negative bacillus **(SELECT 1 DISEASE)**

448. Zinc deficiency **(SELECT 1 DISEASE)**

449. Autosomal dominant trait **(SELECT 1 DISEASE)**

450. Violaceous or heliotrope hue and edema of the eyelids **(SELECT 1 DISEASE)**

Dermatology

Answers

416.   The answer is D. *(Lynch, 3/e, pp 67–68, 122–126, 138–140, 320–324.)* This history is classic for scabies. Contact dermatitis is unlikely in this location and cutaneous larva migrans typically presents with large erythematous, serpiginous tracts. Lesions of dermatitis herpetiformis can appear in the intertriginous area, but there are no burrows and the infection is often associated with a gluten-sensitive enteropathy. Impetigo is an infectious skin disease seen most frequently on the face; it is characterized by discrete vesicles that rupture and form a yellowish crust.

417.   The answer is B. *(Lynch, 3/e, pp 67, 287–291.)* This history is most consistent with tinea capitis that involves a *Microsporum* species. The condition can usually be differentiated from other scalp disorders by its characteristic appearance. Although tinea capitis has different appearances according to the organism that causes the infection, the most common forms are those caused by a *Microsporum* species. Wood's lamp and KOH preparation are useful laboratory methods for diagnosis. Although the condition can resolve spontaneously, therapy should consist of a systemic antifungal agent, such as griseofulvin.

418.   The answer is C. *(Lynch, 3/e, pp 279–285.)* Psoriasis is a fairly common skin disorder that affects 2 to 3 percent of some populations. It occurs equally in both sexes, and most commonly is diagnosed in the third decade of life. Lesions can vary from small pinpoints to plaques that cover large portions of the body. Nail changes are common and include pitting, onychodystrophy, and a yellow-to-brown discoloration ("oil spot"). Auspitz's sign (pinpoint spots of bleeding seen when scales are lifted up off the skin) is a specific feature of psoriasis and can be used to differentiate it from other diseases with a similar appearance.

419.   The answer is E. *(Lynch, 3/e, pp 386–389.)* When evaluating skin lesions for the possibility of malignancy, one can use the mnemonic aid *ABCD: A,* asymmetry (irregular shapes are consistent with malignant lesions); *B,* irregular borders; *C,* variable coloration; *D,* diameter > 7 mm.

420. The answer is C. *(Lynch, 3/e, pp 138–140.)* Impetigo is typically caused by *Staphylococcus aureus* or ß-hemolytic streptococci and usually occurs in children but can occur in adults as well. Many of the strains that cause impetigo are nephritogenic and can result in acute glomerulonephritis. Treatment is with antibiotics, preferably a penicillinase-resistant drug, as many strains are ß-lactamase-positive. The lesions of staphylococcal scalded-skin syndrome are usually sterile.

421. The answer is B. *(Isselbacher, 13/e, p 572.)* Erysipeloid occurs in persons employed as fish or meat handlers. The causative organism is *Erysipelothrix rhusiopathiae*. Arthritis and endocarditis can occur as a result of infection, as well as a septicemia. The most common manifestation is that of a localized violaceous or purple lesion that spreads peripherally with a clearing center. There is a lack of constitutional symptoms, which differentiates erysipeloid from erysipelas.

422. The answer is D. *(Isselbacher, 13/e, pp 303, 557, 725, 864.)* This is a classic presentation for sporotrichosis. The organism, *Sporothrix schenckii*, is found in the soil and can occur as a pulmonary infection or as a systemic disease, but these presentations are unusual. The lesion first begins as a painless, unfixed nodule that eventually becomes fixed and necrotic, the sporotrichotic chancre. A few weeks following the initial lesion there can be sequential formation of multiple nodules along lymphatic channels, which results in "pipestem lymphatics"; however, lymph node involvement is rare. Infection is best treated with potassium iodide.

423. The answer is C. *(Lynch, 3/e, pp 113–117.)* Herpes zoster typically presents with a history of pain, tingling, or itching of the affected area followed by an eruption of vesicles overlying an erythematous base. Although the disease can disseminate and produce diffuse eruptions, it typically presents with involvement of a single dermatome. The disease is not limited to adults and can even be seen in very young children.

424. The answer is E. *(Lynch, 3/e, pp 186–188.)* Molluscum contagiosum is a common benign disease caused by a poxvirus of the same name. The lesions begin as minute papules and can be as large as 3 cm. Lesions can be located on any area of the skin, are usually grouped into one or two small areas, and are limited to less than 20 in number. Diagnosis rests on the characteristic appearance of the lesions, but stained smears of the expressed core and biopsy are definitive. Although they can be pruritic, these lesions are usually asymptomatic and will resolve spontaneously. Freezing or removal with a curette is also effective.

425. The answer is D. *(Lynch, 3/e, p 94, 344.)* Nummular (coin-shaped) eczema appears as a mild to severely pruritic lesion. It initially erupts as minute vesicles and papules that are uniform throughout, but they may later clear centrally and resemble a fungal infection. Lesions are most commonly located on the lower extremities and occur more frequently in men. Treatment consists of hydration of the skin, coal tar, and topical steroids. Follicular eczema is seen in atopic dermatitis.

426. The answer is C. *(Isselbacher, 13/e, pp 304, 1869. Lynch, 3/e, pp 249–250.)* Capillary hemangiomas represent a proliferation of endothelial cells and vascular spaces that are incomplete or small. They present as a small, red nodule that may grow to many centimeters in diameter. The lesions will typically resolve on their own and thus require no treatment, but lesions on exposed areas can bleed secondary to trauma and thus require protective measures.

427. The answer is B. *(Lynch, 3/e, pp 134, 139, 253, 259.)* Staphylococcal scalded-skin syndrome (SSSS) is caused by a *Staphylococcus aureus* strain that produces an epidermolysin that results in a diffuse exfoliation. Although it usually appears in young children, it can also occur in immunocompromised adults. SSSS is limited to the upper epidermis.

428. The answer is E. *(Lynch, 3/e, pp 93, 235.)* Spider angiomas are associated with liver disease. Janeway's lesions are petechial lesions on the palms, and Osler's nodes are painful erythematous nodules located on the fingers and toes. All of these lesions are considered to be due to microvascular embolic phenomena.

429. The answer is E. *(Lynch, 3/e, pp 41, 67, 142, 200, 403.)* Porphyria cutanea tarda is a metabolic disorder that results from a defect or inhibition of the hepatic enzyme uroporphyrinogen decarboxylase. Both ethanol and estrogen are considered to be etiologic agents, with the latter contributing to the current increase in incidence in women. Cutaneous manifestations most commonly present as blistering and fragility of sun-exposed skin that may heal with milia and scar formation. Other cutaneous lesions include scarring alopecia, dystrophic calcification, and scleroderma-like lesions. Diseases associated with this disorder include diabetes mellitus, lupus erythematosus, and hepatitis.

430. The answer is B. *(Lynch, 3/e, pp 275–277.)* Lichen planus is a papulosquamous disorder that typically occurs in adults. The etiology is unknown; however, viruses, genetic factors, and drug reactions are some of the possible causes. The disease can occur locally or be widespread. The lesions occur as pruritic, flat-topped, pink-to-violet papules and involved regions include the flexor forearms, medial thighs, neck, buccal mucosa, and glans penis. Many patients show a positive Koebner's reaction, which is the development of psoriasis in an area of injured skin. Nail changes include ridging, splitting, and pterygium formation. Treatment is usually symptomatic with spontaneous resolution typically occurring in 6 to 18 months, although the disease can last as long as 8 to 9 years.

431. The answer is E. *(Lynch, 3/e, p 263.)* Erythema chronicum migrans is the characteristic rash that develops in a few days to weeks following a tick bite. The rash differs from that of erythema marginatum, which occurs in rheumatic fever, in that there is only a solitary lesion, and it enlarges over a period of days instead of hours. Neurologic, cardiac (AV block, myocarditis), and joint disease can occur. The infective organism is a spirochete *(Borrelia burgdorferi)* and is transmitted by the bite of a tick (e.g., *Ixodes dammini*). Most patients, however, do not remember the bite because ixodid ticks are extremely small. There is resolution in days with proper antibiotic therapy.

432. The answer is C. *(Bialecki, J Am Acad Dermatol 21:891–903, 1989.)* The incidence of measles has decreased greatly since the introduction of a vaccine in 1963. Outbreaks continue to occur and are typically in the spring. Measles is caused by a paramyxovirus spread by droplet infection. The exanthem is an erythematous, maculopapular rash that begins on the face and progresses downward. The lesions tend to develop a brownish color during resolution. Complications can involve the CNS and include a postinfectious encephalomyelitis and, rarely, subacute sclerosing panencephalitis.

433. The answer is D. *(Isselbacher, 13/e, pp 1899–1902.)* Hypersecretion of growth hormone after epiphyseal fusion produces leathery skin, increased hand and foot size, and increased sweating. It may also lead to hypertrophic arthropathy, peripheral neuropathy, and generalized visceromegaly. The clinical features of acromegaly are distinct from those of other diseases; thus, it is readily diagnosed by observation.

434. The answer is A. *(Isselbacher, 13/e, pp 1940–1941.)* Classic hypothyroidism is readily detected by a thorough history and physical examination. Chronic renal disease may also present with a picture of edema and hypothermia that closely resembles hypothyroidism. It may therefore be useful to perform laboratory tests on these patients to determine the possible coexistence of renal disease and hypothyroidism.

435. The answer is A. *(Isselbacher, 13/e, pp 817–818.)* Reye's syndrome is a sometimes-fatal sequela to certain viral illnesses. It presents as an encephalopathy with fatty infiltration and dysfunction of the liver. Salicylates are suspected of potentiating this syndrome; however, they are not believed to be the primary cause.

436. The answer is B. *(Isselbacher, 13/e, pp 272, 561–563.)* Impetigo is a contagious staphylococcal or streptococcal infection of the epidermis. It presents initially as a vesicle or bulla, which ruptures to generate a honey-colored, crusted exudate. Cellulitis may also be caused by staphylococcus or streptococcus, but entails a dermal or subcutaneous infection that presents as a hot, tender, and erythematous region of skin without an exudate. Miliaria, or "prickly heat," is a macular rash caused by occlusion of sweat ducts. Seborrheic dermatitis, or "cradle cap," is a scaly, erythematous lesion that may also be crusted but is generally localized to the scalp and intertriginous areas.

437–441. The answers are 437-C, 438-B, 439-D, 440-A, 441-E. *(Isselbacher, 13/e, p 1723. Lynch, 3/e, p 371.)* Koilonychia, or spoon nails, refers to a nail that is concave in shape. This occurs in iron deficiency anemia, Plummer-Vinson syndrome, and hemochromatosis. Terry's nails are white at the proximal and middle portions, but are pink at the distal ends, and are associated with some forms of hepatic cirrhosis. Though pitting can occur as a normal variant, it is much more pronounced in patients with psoriasis. Half-and-half nails, associated with renal disease and azotemia, present with a white proximal half and a pink or brown distal half. Clubbing of slow onset is associated with chronic respiratory infections, and acute clubbing can occur with lung carcinoma. In children, clubbing can be a sign of congenital heart disease, and in adults it may be associated with gastrointestinal and cardiac disease.

442–445. The answers are 442-C, 443-A, 444-B, 445-A,E. *(Isselbacher, 13/e, pp A1–12, 291, 912–913. Lynch, 3/e, p 364.)* Alopecia areata is an acute onset of hair loss possibly due to autoimmune mechanisms. It presents with smooth, round patterns of hair loss, but there is no inflammation of the affected skin. The disorder can progress to alopecia totalis (whole scalp) or alopecia universalis (whole body). Recurrence is common, and sometimes no regrowth occurs at all. Androgenetic alopecia is very common and occurs in both men and women. Onset usually occurs in the second and third decades, and the pattern of loss varies from family to family, with frontotemporal and vertex loss occurring most often. Women usually present with a diffuse hair loss. Telogen effluvium occurs following pregnancy or stressful events and results from a large percentage of the hair entering telogen phase simultaneously. The hair falls out 1 to 4 months later and this is usually followed by regrowth. Trichotillomania results from a compulsive pulling or twisting of the hair. It occurs as a habit in children but may be the result of a psychologic disturbance in adults.

446–450. The answers are 446-C, 447-D, 448-A, 449-E, 450-B. *(Isselbacher, 13/e, A1–11, A4–54, A6–71, 272, 277, 290, 541, 654, 729, 746, 1566, 2339, 2379–2383.)* Pityriasis rosea is an acute, self-limited disease that typically occurs in young adults. Usually the onset is sudden, without other symptoms such as fever and malaise. The initial lesion is the herald patch, a solitary, oval, annular lesion that is 2 to 6 cm in diameter and is found on the trunk and proximal extremities. This is followed several weeks later by an eruption of small lesions that occur on the same areas and are usually oriented parallel to lines of cleavage ("Christmas tree" pattern). These lesions have a wrinkled center and a scaly border and are hyperpigmented or salmon-pink in appearance. Shingles, tinea corporis, and psoriasis should be ruled out. The disease usually resolves spontaneously in 6 to 8 weeks, and treatment is usually symptomatic.

Chancroid is a sexually transmitted disease that is most often seen in tropical and subtropical areas. Though the organism can be identified from a smear of serous exudate obtained from the border of the lesion by aspiration of a bubo, the organism has fastidious growth requirements and cannot be grown on plain nutrient agar. The lesion is painful, which differentiates it from the chancre of syphilis. The disease can coexist with other venereal diseases, and thus diagnosis rests on the recognition of the clinical features and negative tests for syphilis. Erythromycin is the current drug of choice for treatment.

Acrodermatitis enteropathica usually occurs in infants as an autosomal recessive disorder. The same features of the disease can occur in adults who are receiving TPN that is not supplemented with zinc. Lesions typically occur around the mouth, genitalia, anus, feet, elbows, hands, and knees and consist of erythematous pustules and scales; chronic lesions often resemble those of psoriasis. The diagnosis can be confirmed by measuring plasma zinc levels. Treatment is with zinc supplementation.

Neurofibromatosis, or von Recklinghausen's disease, occurs mostly as an autosomal dominant disorder, although spontaneous mutations are believed to occur. The café au lait spots of neurofibromatosis number at least one in 95 percent of cases and more than six in no less than 78 percent. It should also be noted that patients with more than six lesions that measure 1.5 cm or greater nearly always prove to have the disease. Other cutaneous manifestations include multiple cutaneous tumors. They are quite soft, can measure up to 1 cm or more, occur in many forms (sessile, flattened, pedunculated), and appear flesh-colored or violaceous. Malignant degeneration occurs in a small number.

Dermatomyositis is an acquired inflammatory disease that affects the skin and striated muscle. Major clinical findings include progressive muscle weakness with myalgias and eventual atrophy, and cutaneous manifestations include hyperkeratotic cuticles, periungual telangiectasias, and the pathognomonic finding of flat-topped violaceous papules over the knuckles (Gottron's papules). A heliotrope or violaceous rash on the eyelids, along with edema of the eyelids, is common. Muscle weakness is the presenting symptom in the majority of cases. Corticosteroids are the mainstay of therapy.

Neurology

DIRECTIONS: Each item below contains a question or incomplete statement followed by suggested responses. Select the **one best** response to each question.

451. All the following statements concerning examination of the cranial nerves are true EXCEPT

(A) stimulation of the nasal mucosa with a cotton wisp is a check for the sensation of a branch of the trigeminal nerve

(B) stimulation with sugar or salt of the posterior two-thirds of the tongue while the tongue is protruded will test the sensory function of a branch of the facial nerve

(C) the elevation of the median raphe in the midline when the patient says "Ah" is performed by the vagus nerve

(D) a protruded tongue will point to the side of the lesion if the hypoglossal nerve is involved

(E) the patient should forcibly elevate or shrug his shoulders against the pressure of the examiner during the examination of the accessory nerve

452. Thorough examination of the optic, oculomotor, trochlear, and abducens nerves would include all the following EXCEPT

(A) examination of visual fields and visual acuity

(B) examination of ocular rotation in the six cardinal directions of gaze

(C) testing of the corneal reflex

(D) testing the ability to converge upon a near point

(E) examination of the fundi

453. All the following statements are correct concerning the Argyll Robertson pupil EXCEPT

(A) it is associated with late syphilis, tabes dorsalis in particular

(B) pupils are small, irregular, and unequal

(C) pupils do not react to accommodation

(D) pupils do not respond properly to mydriatic drugs

(E) the exact location of the lesion is uncertain

454. A 60-year-old woman with diabetes mellitus has been told she has carpal tunnel syndrome. All the following are likely to be found in this patient with carpal tunnel syndrome EXCEPT

(A) she is awakened at night with numbness, tingling, and pain
(B) symptoms often occur while she drives a car
(C) atrophy of the thenar muscles occurs
(D) tapping the palmar aspect of the wrist causes paresthesia in the small finger
(D) paresthesias after 30 s of sustained passive wrist flexion occur

455. All the following statements are correct concerning the Romberg test EXCEPT

(A) the test is positive in tabes dorsalis
(B) when the test is positive, further neurologic examination is required
(C) the patient stands erect with feet together, head erect, and eyes open and is then asked to close his or her eyes
(D) a positive test indicates loss of vestibular function
(E) the test is positive when unsteadiness increases with closure of the eyes

456. All the following statements are correct concerning the appearance of the optic disc during funduscopic examination EXCEPT

(A) most lesions of the optic nerve cause the optic disc to become pale
(B) optic atrophy usually requires 4 to 6 weeks to develop
(C) degeneration of the optic nerve causes the optic disc to become chalk-white with sharp, distinct margins
(D) optic atrophy following papilledema produces a yellow-gray disc with poorly defined borders
(E) the vessels and retina are unaffected by papilledema

457. Which of the following descriptions is appropriate to a muscle power grade of 3 (fair)?

(A) Muscle unable to move joint; palpable contraction of muscle
(B) Muscle unable to move joint with gravity eliminated
(C) Muscle unable to overcome resistance other than gravity
(D) Joint moved through range of motion against gravity and some resistance
(E) Joint moved through range of motion overcoming the normal amount of resistance for the muscle

458. Which of the following motor functions is correctly paired with the appropriate nerve root innervation?

(A) Hip adduction, L5
(B) Knee extension, L1
(C) Knee flexion, L3
(D) Great toe extension, L5
(E) Great toe flexion, L4

459. A 28-year-old woman presents complaining that she feels tired when chewing food. Further questioning reveals intermittent diplopia. The most likely diagnosis to pursue is

(A) muscular dystrophy
(B) thyrotoxicosis
(C) myasthenia gravis
(D) multiple sclerosis
(E) primary aldosteronism

460. A 60-year-old man presents with a history of stomping his feet as he walks. The patient also has noticed that he continually hits things with his feet accidentally. Physical examination reveals loss of vibratory and position sense without loss of pain or temperature perception. The most likely diagnosis is

(A) lesion of the medulla
(B) anterior spinal artery syndrome
(C) posterior column syndrome
(D) lesion of the thalamic nucleus ventralis posterolateralis
(E) syringomyelic syndrome

461. All the following would be found in a patient with Duchenne's muscular dystrophy EXCEPT

(A) dorsal shift of the upper trunk
(B) atrophy of calf muscles
(C) difficulty with stair climbing
(D) circumduction during the swing phase of gait
(E) a positive Meryon's sign

462. Which of the following statements is correct concerning reflex eye movements?

(A) Oculocephalic, or "doll's eye," reflex is elicited by slowly moving the head from side to side
(B) If the brainstem is intact, comatose patients' eyes should move conjugately in the same direction that the head is turned
(C) In comatose patients with brainstem involvement, the eyes always move dysconjugately or not at all
(D) If the brainstem is intact, the oculovestibular, or caloric, reflex test, which introduces ice-cold water into the external auditory canal, produces tonic deviation of the eyes to the side opposite that of irrigation
(E) The oculovestibular, or caloric, reflex is not used to assess brainstem involvement

463. A patient presents complaining of complete loss of vision. Physical examination shows pupillary light reflexes and eye movements intact. Funduscopic examination is unremarkable. The most likely explanation is

(A) bilateral lesions of the occipital lobes

(B) lesion of one occipital lobe

(C) enucleation of the eyes

(D) bilateral lesions of the striate cortex below the calcarine fissure

(E) bilateral severance of the optic nerves

DIRECTIONS: Each group of questions below consists of lettered options followed by numbered items. For each numbered item, select the appropriate lettered option(s). Each lettered option may be used once, more than once, or not at all. **Choose exactly the number of options indicated following each item.**

Items 464–468

A 26-year-old man presents to the emergency room after a high speed motor vehicle accident. Match the following findings.

(A) Deltoid and biceps motor function is intact; extensor carpi radialis longus and brevis muscles are not functional
(B) Flexion of the distal interphalangeal joints is intact; finger adduction and abduction is not functional
(C) Sensation is intact over and just inferior to the clavicle; sensation is not intact over the lateral aspect of the shoulder and deltoid region
(D) Sensation is not intact below the nipple line except for preserved perianal sensation
(E) The anal sphincter is flaccid when the glans penis is squeezed

464. The lowest functioning neurologic level is C4 **(SELECT 1 FINDING)**

465. The lowest functioning neurologic level is C5 **(SELECT 1 FINDING)**

466. The lowest functioning neurologic level is C8 **(SELECT 1 FINDING)**

467. The lesion is incomplete and some neurologic recovery is likely to occur **(SELECT 1 FINDING)**

468. The patient is in spinal shock **(SELECT 1 FINDING)**

Items 469–472

Match the visual-field defects below with the causative lesion.

(A) Lesion behind the optic chiasm
(B) Lesion in the lower fibers of the geniculocalcarine pathway
(C) Lesion of the calcarine cortex
(D) Lesion of the optic chiasm
(E) Lesion of the tip of an occipital lobe

469. Upper homonymous quadrantanopia **(SELECT 1 LESION)**

470. Homonymous hemianopia with macular sparing **(SELECT 1 LESION)**

471. Complete homonymous hemianopia **(SELECT 1 LESION)**

472. Bitemporal hemianopia **(SELECT 1 LESION)**

Items 473–476

Match the signs and symptoms below with the appropriate disorder.

- (A) Chronic proximal progressive spinal muscular atrophy
- (B) Progressive spinal muscular atrophy
- (C) Progressive bulbar palsy
- (D) Primary lateral sclerosis
- (E) Amyotrophic lateral sclerosis

473. Weakness of the muscles of the jaw, face, tongue, pharynx, and larynx resulting in difficulties with articulation and mastication **(SELECT 1 DISORDER)**

474. Stiffness of the fingers associated with weakness of the hand, followed by atrophic weakness of the hands and forearms, slight spasticity of the legs, and generalized hyperreflexia **(SELECT 1 DISORDER)**

475. Symmetric weakness and atrophy of the pelvic girdle and proximal leg muscles; later involvement of the shoulder girdle and upper arm muscles; finally, involvement of the distal limbs and absence of tendon reflexes **(SELECT 1 DISORDER)**

476. Symmetric wasting of the intrinsic hand muscles, slowly progressing to more proximal muscles of the arms; diminished or absent tendon reflexes **(SELECT 1 DISORDER)**

Items 477–480

Match the descriptions below with the correct gait.

- (A) Ataxic gait
- (B) Hemiplegic gait
- (C) Parkinsonian gait
- (D) Spastic gait
- (E) Steppage gait

477. The upper torso is slightly stooped forward; the feet shuffle with loss of arm swing **(SELECT 1 GAIT)**

478. The limb affected with footdrop is lifted higher than normal **(SELECT 1 GAIT)**

479. The feet are widely spaced; steps occur with the foot lifted abruptly and too high and brought down in a stamping manner **(SELECT 1 GAIT)**

480. The affected limb is moved forward by abduction and circumduction **(SELECT 1 GAIT)**

Items 481–483

Match each patient with the probable injury.

(A) Median nerve injury at
    the wrist
(B) Median nerve injury at
    the elbow
(C) Ulnar nerve injury at
    the wrist
(D) Ulnar nerve injury at
    the elbow

(E) Posterior interosseus nerve
    injury at the proximal
    forearm
(F) Radial nerve injury at
    the arm
(G) Ulnar nerve injury at
    the arm

481. A 22-year-old man has two-point discrimination of 12 mm at the index finger and is unable to make the "OK" sign **(SELECT 1 INJURY)**

482. A 17-year-old woman has very dry skin of the small finger. All fingers wrinkle when placed in water except the small finger. She has weak abduction of the index finger and strong flexion of the distal inter-phalangeal joint of the small finger. She can extend the wrist but is unable to extend the digits. Wrist extension results in radial deviation. **(SELECT 2 INJURIES)**

483. A 50-year-old woman complains of weakness of wrist extension and numbness on the dorsum of the thumb after a humeral fracture **(SELECT 1 INJURY)**

Items 484–488

Match each patient with the likely clinical findings.

(A) Perianal sensory loss
(B) Posterior calf sensory loss
(C) Plantar foot sensory loss
(D) Lateral calf sensory loss
(E) Dorsal foot sensory loss

(F) Medial calf sensory loss
(G) Anterior thigh sensory loss
(H) Hip flexor weakness
(I) Quadriceps weakness
(J) Extensor digitorum longus
    weakness
(K) Gastrocnemius weakness

484. A 20-year-old patient with an L4-L5 disk injury **(SELECT 3 FINDINGS)**

485. A 50-year-old patient with L2 nerve root loss **(SELECT 2 FINDINGS)**

486. A 60-year-old patient with L3-L4 disk injury **(SELECT 2 FINDINGS)**

487. A 70-year-old patient with S1 nerve root loss **(SELECT 3 FINDINGS)**

488. A 17-year-old patient with S2-S4 nerve root loss **(SELECT 1 FINDING)**

DIRECTIONS: Each group of questions below consists of four lettered options followed by a set of numbered items. For each numbered item select

A	if the item is associated with	(A) only
B	if the item is associated with	(B) only
C	if the item is associated with	**both** (A) and (B)
D	if the item is associated with	**neither** (A) nor (B)

Each lettered option may be used **once, more than once, or not at all.**

Items 489–492

(A) Vascular claudication
(B) Neurogenic claudication
(C) Both
(D) Neither

489. Pain with walking

490. Pain relieved with standing

491. Pain that consistently correlates with amount of exercise

492. Positive stoop test

Items 493–496

(A) Asterixis
(B) Myoclonus
(C) Both
(D) Neither

493. Rhythmic movement

494. Involvement of the upper extremities

495. Sudden relaxation of a muscle group

496. Sudden contraction of a muscle group

Items 497–500

(A) Essential tremor
(B) Parkinsonian tremor
(C) Both
(D) Neither

497. Occurrence at rest

498. Intensification at the termination of movement

499. Association with increased muscle tone

500. Increase with fatigue or fright

Neurology

Answers

451. The answer is B. *(Seidel, 3/e, pp 735–741.)* Stimulation of the anterior two-thirds of the protruded tongue with sugar, salt, tartaric acid, or similar substances will test the peripheral branches of the facial nerve, the lingual nerve, and the chorda tympani. A small amount of the test substance is placed on one side of the tongue and identified by the patient before the tongue is drawn into the mouth so that diffusion of the taste to other areas of the tongue is prevented. Stimulation of the nasal mucosa with a wisp of cotton tests the sensation of the nasociliary division of the ophthalmic branch of the trigeminal nerve. Examination of the vagus nerve can be performed by examining the elevation of the median raphe in the midline while the patient says "Ah." If a lesion involves the hypoglossal nerve, the protruded tongue will deviate to the side of the lesion. To test the integrity of the accessory nerve, the examiner should palpate the movement of both upper trapezius muscles and attempt to depress the shoulders while the patient forcibly shrugs his shoulders against this resistance; to test the lower portion of the accessory nerve, the patient should brace his shoulders backward and down.

452. The answer is C. *(Seidel, 3/e, pp 736–739.)* The corneal reflex is a function of the ophthalmic division of the trigeminal nerve. Examination of the optic nerve should include visual fields, visual acuity, and inspection of the retina and optic nerve head with the aid of an ophthalmoscope. The examination of the oculomotor, trochlear, and abducens nerves involves ocular rotation through the six cardinal directions of gaze as well as convergence upon a near point.

453. The answer is C. *(Adams, 5/e, p 243.)* The Argyll Robertson pupil, which is small, irregular, and unequal, is associated with chronic and late syphilis, particularly tabes dorsalis. The pupil fails to react to light, but does react to accommodation. It does not respond normally to mydriatic drugs. The exact location of the lesion is not known.

454. The answer is D. *(American Society for Surgery of the Hand, 3/e, p 91.)* Carpal tunnel syndrome results from compression of the median nerve as it passes through the carpal tunnel. Patients have numbness, tingling, and pain in the distribution of the median nerve: thumb, index, long, and ring fingers. The small finger is usually not involved. This finding does not, however, exclude the diagnosis. Symptoms often awaken the patient at night. Symptoms may become worse with certain activities such as driving a car or reading a newspaper. Repetitive activities involving the hands and wrists may also cause symptoms. It is often bilateral and more common in women. Carpal tunnel syndrome is associated with pregnancy, diabetes mellitus, and thyroid disease; most cases, however, have no associated systemic disease. Long-standing cases may result in atrophy of the thenar muscles. Symptoms may be reproduced by tapping the volar aspect of the wrist over the median nerve (Tinel's sign) or by passively flexing the wrist for up to 1 min (Phalen's test).

455. The answer is D. *(Seidel, 3/e, p 298.)* The Romberg test is performed by having the patient stand with feet together, head erect, and eyes open. The patient is examined for steadiness and then asked to close his or her eyes. A positive test occurs when the patient displays increased unsteadiness with eyes closed. The Romberg test is not specific, does not assess vestibular function, and requires further neurologic assessment to determine the lesion responsible. The test is positive in patients with tabes dorsalis.

456. The answer is E. *(Seidel, 3/e, pp 252–253, 727.)* Most diseases that affect the optic nerve cause the optic disc to become pale; this usually occurs over 4 to 6 weeks. Degeneration of the optic nerve (as caused by multiple sclerosis, tumor of the nerve, or traumatic transection) results in a chalk-white disc with distinct margins. However, if atrophy is the result of papilledema or papillitis, then the disc develops a yellow-gray color and the margins become irregular and indistinct. The adjacent retina becomes altered and the vessels are also affected.

457. The answer is C. *(Evarts, 2/e, p 17.)* A commonly accepted means of grading muscle strength is as follows:

Grade 0. No motion of joint with gravity eliminated and no palpable contraction of muscle are produced.

Grade 1 (Trace). The muscle is unable to move the joint with gravity eliminated, and palpable contraction of muscle can be detected.

Grade 2 (Poor). Motion of the joint can be produced if gravity is removed but motion cannot be produced against gravity.

Grade 3 (Fair). The muscle can move joint through full range of motion against gravity but cannot overcome any additional resistance.

Grade 4 (Good). The joint can be moved through a range of motion against gravity and some resistance but is not able to overcome the same amount of resistance that the unaffected contralateral muscle is able to overcome.

Grade 5 (Normal). The joint can be moved through a range of motion while it overcomes a normal amount of resistance.

458. The answer is D. *(Rockwood, 4/e, p 1533.)* A careful evaluation of motor function allows the examining physician to determine the level of spinal cord injury or the level of nerve root involvement. The following motor functions and their respective nerve root innervations should be evaluated: hip adduction, L1-L2; knee extension, L3-L4; knee flexion, L5-S1; great toe extension, L5; great toe flexion, S1.

459. The answer is C. *(Mayo Clinic, 6/e, pp 468–470, 477–480.)* Myasthenia gravis is a muscular weakness that occurs when repetitive use of a muscle results in exhaustion of its contractile power; although a progressive paresis results, rest partially restores muscle strength. Usually the muscles of the eyes and, slightly less commonly, of the jaw, throat, face, and neck are the first to be affected. Muscular dystrophy usually presents by the third year of life with muscle weakness that causes difficulty walking or running and a tendency to fall. Thyrotoxicosis has been associated with periodic paralysis mainly in young males of Japanese and Chinese descent; the periodic paralysis is unrelated to the severity of the thyrotoxicosis. Patients with multiple sclerosis present with weakness of one or more limbs almost 50 percent of the time. Hypokalemic weakness can result from the hypersecretion of aldosterone in primary aldosteronism.

460. The answer is C. *(Adams, 6/e, pp 162–163.)* The patient who has a lesion of the posterior column will have a loss of the position and vibratory sense below the level of the lesion, but pain and temperature sensation remain intact or only mildly affected. Lesions of the medulla produce a crossed disturbance consisting of a loss of pain and temperature sensation on one side of the face and the opposite side of the body. This pattern is due to a lateral medullary infarction that affects the trigeminal tract or nucleus and the lateral spinothalamic tract. Infarction of the anterior spinal artery will produce motor paralysis and loss of pain and temperature sensation below the lesion with relative or absolute sparing of proprioception; the lesion often affects the ventral part of the cord and the corticospinal tracts along with the ventral gray matter. A lesion of the nucleus ventralis posterolateralis of the thalamus is most often vascular, although tumor is a possibility. The lesion results in loss or deterioration of all forms of sensation on the opposite side of the body; however, position sense is often more profoundly affected than others. A very high lesion of the central gray matter will affect the fibers conducting pain and temperature as they cross the cord in the anterior commissure; this will affect several dermatomes on one or both sides, but will spare tactile sensation. Syringomyelia is the most common cause of such a lesion.

461. The answer is B. *(Mayo Clinic, 6/e, pp 410, 480. Morrissy, 4/e, pp 410–411.)* Duchenne's muscular dystrophy is a disease primarily of males that usually becomes evident between the ages of 18 and 36 months. Affected children have symmetric weakness of the pelvic girdle followed by involvement of the shoulder girdle muscles 3 to 5 years later. The patients may shift the upper trunk in a dorsal direction to compensate for weakness of the gluteus maximus. Pseudohypertrophy of the calves (not atrophy) occurs because of weak proximal muscles. The child has difficulty climbing stairs and may circumduct during the swing phase of gait. When the child with weakness of the shoulder girdle is picked up by the examiner's hands under the child's arms, the child slides through the examiner's hands, which is a positive Meryon's sign. The child may arise by pushing off of the legs with the upper extremities to compensate for weakness of the quadriceps and gluteus maximus, which is Gowers' sign.

462.   The answer is C. *(Mayo Clinic, 6/e, pp 142–145, 294–295.)* The oculocephalic, or "doll's eye," reflex is performed by rapidly rotating the head from side to side; if the brainstem is intact in a comatose patient, then the eyes will move conjugately in the direction opposite the rotation of the head. If the brainstem is not intact, then the eyes will move dysconjugately or not at all. The oculovestibular, or caloric, reflex is performed by applying ice-cold water into the external auditory canal; the comatose patient with an intact brainstem will respond with tonic deviation of the eyes to the side of irrigation. If the brainstem function is not intact, then the reflex will be absent or the eyes will move dysconjugately.

463.   The answer is A. *(Adams, 6/e, pp 460–464.)* Bilateral lesions of the occipital lobes, with destruction of area 17, will result in loss of sight. The pupillary reflexes will be intact because their fibers terminate in the midbrain. Complete interruption of the optic nerves would result in a lack of pupillary reflexes in addition to blindness. Enucleation of the eyes would also result in a lack of pupillary reflexes. Lesions of the striate cortex below the calcarine fissure result in upper-quadrant field defects caused by damage of the fibers from the lower half of the retina. A lesion of one occipital lobe would not result in complete loss of vision.

464–468.   The answers are 464-C, 465-A, 466-B, 467-D, 468-E. *(Mayo Clinic, 6/e, p 250. Rockwood, 4/e, pp 1250–1255.)* In the patient who presents with a neurologic deficit, a careful sensory and motor examination will determine the approximate level of spinal cord injury. The sensory examination can be performed by documentation of intact sharp versus dull sensation. There is, however, overlap and variation of the sensory dermatomes. The following can be used as a guide to the examination of the sensory dermatomes of the cervical nerves: C2, back of the scalp; C3, anterior aspect of the neck; C4, lateral and inferior areas over the clavicle; C5, lateral deltoid area; C6, radial aspect of thumb; C7, middle finger; C8, ulnar border of small finger.

If sensation is intact at any level below the level of injury, the lesion is classified as incomplete, and some neurologic recovery is likely to occur. Preserved perianal sensation may be the only evidence of an incomplete lesion.

After completion of the sensory examination, a motor examination is carried out by evaluating sequential nerve root levels. The following can be used as a guide for cervical nerve root evaluation: C5, deltoid and biceps; C6, extensor carpi radialis longus and brevis; C7, triceps and finger extensors; C8, finger flexors; T1, intrinsic muscles of the hand.

The bulbocavernous reflex is a simple sensory-motor pathway that functions even with disruption of spinal cord function above. This reflex is intact if contraction of the anal sphincter (on the examiner's gloved finger) results from a squeeze on the glans penis, tap on the mons pubis, or tug on the urethral catheter. If this reflex is absent, the patient is in spinal shock and a permanent complete lesion cannot be diagnosed with certainty. Spinal shock usually resolves within 24 h and the bulbocavernous reflex returns. If there is no sensory or motor sparing below the level of injury and the bulbocavernous reflex is present, the lesion is complete and no recovery of motor function can be expected.

469–472. The answers are 469-B, 470-C, 471-A, 472-D. *(Adams, 6/e, pp 253–255.)* A lesion of the lower fibers of the geniculocalcarine pathway (Flechsig's, Meyer's, or Archambault's loop) will cause a defect of the upper quadrants of the contralateral visual fields or an upper homonymous quadrantanopia. A lesion that completely destroys the calcarine cortex will cause a complete homonymous hemianopia, but often the macula is spared owing to the fact that some of the macular fibers terminate in the ipsilateral striate cortex. A complete homonymous hemianopia indicates that the lesion lies in the visual pathway behind the optic chiasm, but it is not localizing; only incomplete homonymous hemianopia will aid the examiner in localizing the lesion. A lesion interrupting the decussating fibers of the optic chiasm results in a bitemporal hemianopia.

473–476. The answers are 473-C, 474-E, 475-A, 476-B. *(Adams, 6/e, pp 1089–1094, 1454–1457.)* Progressive bulbar palsy shows prominent symptoms related to weakness of the muscles innervated by the motor nuclei of the lower brainstem. Weakness of the muscles of the face, tongue, jaw, pharynx, and larynx results in difficulty with articulation and mastication; fasciculations and focal tissue loss of the tongue are seen early.

Amyotrophic lateral sclerosis typically presents with decreased function of a hand associated with stiffness of the fingers and awkwardness of fine finger movements. Over a period of months the triad of atrophic weakness of the hands and forearms, slight spasticity of the legs, and generalized hyper-reflexia occurs; there is no loss of sensory function.

Chronic proximal progressive spinal muscle atrophy begins with symmetric weakness of the pelvic girdle and proximal leg muscles of young children, one-third before 2 years of age and one-half from ages 3 to 8 years. The shoulder girdle and upper arm muscles become involved next; this is followed by involvement of the distal limb muscles and loss of tendon reflexes.

Progressive spinal muscular atrophy is a symmetric wasting of the intrinsic hand muscles, which slowly progresses to the proximal parts of the arm. The legs and thighs are less often the sites of atrophic weakness. The tendon reflexes are diminished or absent.

477–480. The answers are 477-C, 478-E, 479-A, 480-B. *(Mayo Clinic, 6/e, pp 170–173, 312, 314.)* Ataxic gait, often characterized by clumsiness, occurs when the patient places his feet widely apart and when taking steps lifts the advancing foot high. The foot is then brought down in a slapping or stamping manner.

Hemiplegic gait is the result of increased muscle tone and spasticity of the involved limb with downward flexion of the toe. The limb is moved forward by abduction and circumduction. Because of the flexion of the toe, the shoe of the affected limb will show increased wear along the outer aspect.

Parkinsonian gait is noted for the forward stoop of the head and shoulders, with arms slightly abducted and forearms partially flexed; there is decreased arm swing as the feet shuffle.

Steppage gait occurs in patients with footdrop; the affected foot is raised higher than normal to prevent dragging or stubbing of the toe. Bilateral footdrop results in a gait resembling that of a high-stepping horse.

Spastic gait is a scissorlike movement of the spastic lower limbs in a stiff and jerky manner. Extreme compensatory movements of the trunk and upper extremities are often necessary.

481–483. The answers are 481-B; 482-C,E; 483-F. *(Miller, 2/e, pp 245–248, 435–438.)* Loss of sensory function can be assessed by change in two-point discrimination, loss of skin sweating, or loss of normal skin wrinkle in water. Normal two-point discrimination is approximately 5 mm. This is the minimal distance at which a patient can discriminate two points touched lightly on the pulp of the finger at the same time. Sensory function is best assessed on the pulp of the index finger for median nerve function and the pulp of the small finger for ulnar nerve function. The "OK" sign requires an intact flexor digitorum profundus to the index finger and an intact flexor pollicis longus for flexion of the interphalangeal joint of the thumb. Injury to the anterior interosseous or median nerves will result in loss of the ability to make the "OK" sign. The first dorsal interosseus muscle can be palpated in the first web space when a patient abducts the index finger against resistance. This muscle is supplied by the ulnar nerve. The flexor digitorum profundus to the ring and small fingers is supplied by the ulnar nerve. This muscle is innervated high in the forearm. Therefore, if these muscles are functioning, the injury must be at a lower level. The radial nerve can be injured with fractures of the humerus. The radial nerve supplies wrist extension. Injury to this nerve often results in wristdrop. The radial nerve gives off the posterior interosseous nerve. Injury of this nerve results in loss of extension of all digits and the extensor carpi ulnaris muscle. The brachioradialis and extensor carpi radialis are spared and provide wrist extension. Wrist extension, however results in radial deviation due to loss of the extensor carpi ulnaris muscle.

484–488. The answers are 484-D,E,J; 485-G,H; 486-F,I; 487-B,C,K; 488-A *(Miller, 2/e, p 277.)* Disk pathology will frequently involve characteristic root levels with fairly consistent clinical findings. The following are characteristic findings for lumbar and sacral levels of pathology (EDL=extensor digitorum longus; EHL=extensor hallucis longus).

Level	Nerve Root Affected	Sensory Loss	Motor Loss
L1-L3	L2-L3	anterior thigh	hip flexors
L3-L4	L4	medial calf	quadriceps, tibialis anterior
L4-L5	L5	lateral calf, dorsal foot	EDL, EHL
L5-S1	S1	posterior calf, plantar foot	gastrocnemius
S2-S4	S2-S4	perianal	bowel/bladder

489–492. The answers are 489-C, 490-A, 491-A, 492-B. *(Crenshaw, 8/e, p 3840.)* Spinal stenosis can lead to back, buttock, and thigh and leg pain. The pain is eased with sitting or recumbency and increased with standing and walking. This pain is called *neurogenic claudication* and should be differentiated from vascular claudication. The latter is also brought on by walking but is relieved by standing. The amount of exercise required to bring on symptoms is generally consistent and dependable in vascular claudication. Exercise causes symptoms in vascular claudication, whereas symptoms of neurogenic claudication are brought on by position. A patient with neurogenic claudication, when asked to continue walking or standing after the onset of pain, may assume a stooped position to relieve the symptoms (positive stoop test).

493–496. The answers are 493-D, 494-C, 495-A, 496-B. *(Mayo Clinic, 6/e, p 164–166.)* Asterixis, also known as "wrist flapping," results from the sudden relaxation of the wrist extensors. This movement is arrhythmic and can occur with hepatic failure and diffuse (metabolic) encephalopathies such as uremia and phenytoin (Dilantin) intoxication. Myoclonus is an arrhythmic movement of the extremities (upper or lower) or trunk that results from the sudden contraction of one or more muscle groups.

497–500. The answers are 497-B, 498-A, 499-B, 500-C. *(Mayo Clinic, 6/e, pp 161–162.)* Essential tremor is absent at rest and appears with movements or actions that require support of an extremity. The tremor intensifies at the termination of the movement. Parkinsonian tremor, also referred to as "pill-rolling type," occurs at rest and normally lessens with movement. It is generally associated with increased muscle tone and occurs at a rate of 3 to 6 per second. All types of tremor are increased in response to fatigue or fright.

Bibliography

Adams RD, Victor M, Ropper AH: *Principles of Neurology,* 6/e. New York, McGraw-Hill, 1997.

American Society for Surgery of the Hand: *The Hand: Examination and Diagnosis,* 3/e. New York, Churchill Livingstone, 1990.

Athreya BH, Silverman BK: I East Norwalk, CT, Appleton & Lange, 1985.

Badgett RG, Tanaka DJ, Hunt DK, et al: Can moderate chronic obstructive pulmonary disease be diagnosed by historical and physical findings alone? *Am J Med* 94(2):188–96, 1993.

Bates B, Hoeckelman RA: *A Guide to Physical Examination and History Taking,* 5/e. Philadelphia, Lippincott, 1991.

Behrman RE, Vaughan VC (eds): *Nelson Textbook of Pediatrics,* 15/e. Philadelphia, Saunders, 1995.

Berkow R, Fletcher AJ (eds): *The Merck Manual: General Medicine,* vol 1, 16/e. Rahway, NJ, Merck, 1992.

Bialecki C, et al: The six classic childhood exanthems: A review and update. *J Am Acad Dermatol* 21:891–903, 1989.

Burnside JW, McGlynn TJ: *Physical Diagnosis,* 17/e. Baltimore, Williams & Wilkins, 1987.

Carson WG, Lovell WW, Whitesides TE: Congenital elevation of the scapula. *J Bone Joint Surg* 63A(8):1199–1207, 1981.

Cattau EL, et al: The accuracy of the physical examination in the diagnosis of suspected ascites. *JAMA* 247:1164–1165, 1982.

Chervu A, Clagett GP, Valentine RJ, et al: Role of physical examination in detection of abdominal aortic aneurysms. *Surgery* 117(4):454–7, 1995.

Crenshaw AH (ed): *Campbell's Operative Orthopaedics,* 8/e. St. Louis, Mosby, 1992.

Delp MH, Manning RT: *Major's Physical Diagnosis: An Introduction to the Clinical Process,* 9/e. Philadelphia, Saunders, 1981.

Emergency Cardiac Care Committee and Subcommittees, American Heart Association: Guidelines for cardiopulmonary and emergency cardiac care. *JAMA* 268:2174, 1992.

Eskelinen M, Ikonen J, Lipponen P: The value of history-taking, physical examination and computer assistance in the diagnosis of acute appendicitis in patients more than 50 years old. *Scand J Gastroenterol* 30(4):349–355, 1995.

Evarts CM (ed): *Surgery of the Musculoskeletal System*, 2/e. New York, Churchill Livingstone, 1990.

Gartland JJ: *Fundamentals of Orthopaedics*, 4/e. Philadelphia, Saunders, 1987.

Harvey AM, et al: *The Principles and Practice of Medicine*, 22/e. East Norwalk, CT, Appleton & Lange, 1988.

Hathaway WE, Hay WW, Groothuis JR, et al: *Current Pediatric Diagnosis and Treatment*, 11/e. East Norwalk, CT, Appleton & Lange, 1993.

Hoppenfeld S, Zeide MS: *Orthopaedic Dictionary*. Philadelphia, Lippincott, 1994.

Isselbacher KJ, Braunwald E, Wilson JD, et al (eds): *Harrison's Principles of Internal Medicine*, 13/e. New York, McGraw-Hill, 1994.

Lewis RC, Jr: *Primary Care Orthopaedics*. New York, Churchill Livingstone, 1988.

McCullough DL (ed): *Difficult Diagnoses in Urology*. New York, Churchill Livingstone, 1988.

Lynch PJ: *House Officers Series: Dermatology,* 3/e. Baltimore, Williams & Wilkins, 1994.

Magee DJ: *Orthopedic Physical Assessment*, 2/e. Philadelphia, Saunders, 1992.

Mann RA: The great toe. *Orthop Clin North Am* 20:519–533, 1989.

Markovchick VJ, Pons PT, Wolfe RE: *Emergency Medicine Secrets*. Philadelphia, Hanley & Belfus, 1993.

Mayo Clinic, Department of Neurology: *Clinical Examinations in Neurology*, 6/e. Philadelphia, Saunders, 1991.

Miller MD: *Review of Orthopaedics*, 2/e. Philadelphia, Saunders, 1996.

Miller MD, Cooper DE, Warner JJP: *Review of Sports Medicine and Arthroscopy*. Philadelphia, Saunders, 1995.

Moore KL: *Clinically Oriented Anatomy,* 3/e. Baltimore, Williams & Wilkins, 1992.

Morrey BF (ed): *The Elbow and Its Disorders*, 2/e. Philadelphia, Saunders, 1993.

Morrissy RT, Weinstein SL: *Lovell and Winter's Pediatric Orthopaedics*, 4/e. Philadelphia, Lippincott, 1996.

Munro J, Edwards CRW: *Macleods's Clinical Examination*, 9/e. New York, Churchill Livingstone, 1995.

Muris JW, Starmans R, Wolfs GG, et al: The diagnostic value of rectal examination. *Fam Pract* 10(1):34–37, 1993.

O'Driscoll SW, Morrey BF, Korinek S, An KN: Elbow subluxation and dislocation: A spectrum of instability. *Clin Ortho*p 280:186–197, 1992.

Pansky B: *Review of Gross Anatomy,* 6/e. New York, McGraw-Hill, 1996.

Rockwood CA, Jr, Green DP, Bucholz RW, Heckman JD: *Fractures in Adults*, 4/e. Philadelphia, Lippincott, 1996.

Sapira JD: *The Art and Science of Bedside Diagnosis.* Baltimore, Urban & Schwarzenberg, 1989.

Seidel HM, Ball JW, Dains JE, et al: *Mosby's Guide to Physical Examination,* 3/e. St. Louis, Mosby, 1995.

Simmons BP, Southmayd WW, Risoborough EJ: Congenital radioulnar synostosis. *J Hand Surg* 8:829–838, 1983.

Sullivan D, Warren RF, Pavlov H, et al: Stress fractures in 51 runners. *Clin Orthop* 187:188, 1984.

Talley N, O'Connor S: *Clinical Examination*, 2/e. Philadelphia, Maclennan & Petty, 1992.

Thompson GH, Salter RB: Legg-Calvé-Perthes disease: Current concepts and controversies. *Orthop Clin North Am* 18:617–635, 1987.

Tintinalli JE, Ruiz E, Krome RL: *Emergency Medicine: A Comprehensive Study Guide*, 4/e. New York, McGraw-Hill, 1996.

Torg FS, Conrad W, Kalen V: Clinical diagnosis of anterior cruciate ligament instability in the athlete. *Am J Sports Med* 4:84–93, 1976.

Vaughan D, Asbury T: *General Ophthalmology*, 13/e. East Norwalk, CT, Appleton & Lange, 1992.

Yamamoto M, Hibi H, Miyake K: Role of prostate-specific antigen and digital rectal examination in detection of prostate cancer. *Int J Urol* 1(1):74–77, 1994.

Notes

Notes

ISBN 0-07-052531-5

90000

9 780070 525313